Brain Stimulation in Psychiatric Treatment

Review of Psychiatry Series
John M. Oldham, M.D., M.S.
Michelle B. Riba, M.D., M.S.
Series Editors

Brain Stimulation in Psychiatric Treatment

EDITED BY

Sarah H. Lisanby, M.D.

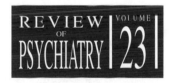

REVIEW OF PSYCHIATRY VOLUME 23

No. 1

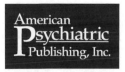

American Psychiatric Publishing, Inc.

Washington, DC
London, England

Copyright © 2004 American Psychiatric Publishing, Inc.
ALL RIGHTS RESERVED

Manufactured in the United States of America on acid-free paper
08 07 06 05 04   5 4 3 2 1
First Edition

Typeset in Adobe's Palatino

American Psychiatric Publishing, Inc.
1000 Wilson Boulevard
Arlington, VA 22209-3901
www.appi.org

The correct citation for this book is
Lisanby SH (editor): *Brain Stimulation in Psychiatric Treatment* (Review of Psychiatry Series, Volume 23; Oldham JM and Riba MB, series editors). Washington, DC, American Psychiatric Publishing, 2004

Library of Congress Cataloging-in-Publication Data
Brain stimulation in psychiatric treatment / edited by Sarah H. Lisanby.
      p. ; cm.—(Review of psychiatry ; v. 23, no. 1)
Includes bibliographical references and index.
ISBN 1-58562-175-7 (pbk. : alk. paper)
      1. Magnetic brain stimulation. 2. Electroconvulsive therapy. 3. Mental illness—Treatment. I. Lisanby, Sarah H., 1965– II. Review of psychiatry series; v. 23, 1.
      [DNLM: 1. Mental Disorders—therapy. 2. Brain—physiopathology. 3. Electroconvulsive Therapy—methods. WM 412 B814 2004]
RC386.6.M32B736 2004
616.89'122—dc22

                                                                    2003065579

British Library Cataloguing in Publication Data
A CIP record is available from the British Library.

Contents

Contributors

Benjamin D. Greenberg, M.D., Ph.D.
Associate Professor, Department of Psychiatry and Human Behavior, Butler Hospital and Brown University School of Medicine, Providence, Rhode Island

Ralph E. Hoffman, M.D.
Associate Professor, Department of Psychiatry, Yale University School of Medicine, New Haven, Connecticut

Markus Kosel, M.D., Ph.D.
Resident, Brain Stimulation Group, Department of Psychiatry, University Hospital, Bonn, Germany

Sarah H. Lisanby, M.D.
Director, Magnetic Brain Stimulation Laboratory, Department of Biological Psychiatry, New York State Psychiatric Institute; Associate Professor of Clinical Psychiatry, Department of Psychiatry, College of Physicians and Surgeons, Columbia University, New York, New York

John M. Oldham, M.D., M.S.
Professor and Chair, Department of Psychiatry and Behavioral Sciences, Medical University of South Carolina, Charleston, South Carolina

Michelle B. Riba, M.D., M.S.
Clinical Professor and Associate Chair for Education and Academic Affairs, Department of Psychiatry, University of Michigan Medical School, Ann Arbor, Michigan

Harold A. Sackeim, Ph.D.
Division Chief, Department of Biological Psychiatry, New York State Psychiatric Institute; Professor of Clinical Psychology in the Departments of Psychiatry and Radiology, College of Physicians and Surgeons, Columbia University, New York, New York

Thomas E. Schlaepfer, M.D.
Professor, Brain Stimulation Group, Department of Psychiatry, University Hospital, Bonn, Germany; Associate Professor, Department of Psychiatry, The Johns Hopkins University School of Medicine, Baltimore, Maryland

Introduction to the Review of Psychiatry Series

John M. Oldham, M.D., M.S.
Michelle B. Riba, M.D., M.S., Series Editors

2004 REVIEW OF PSYCHIATRY SERIES TITLES

- *Developmental Psychobiology*
  EDITED BY B.J. CASEY, PH.D.
- *Neuropsychiatric Assessment*
  EDITED BY STUART C. YUDOFSKY, M.D., AND H. FLORENCE KIM, M.D.
- *Brain Stimulation in Psychiatric Treatment*
  EDITED BY SARAH H. LISANBY, M.D.
- *Cognitive-Behavior Therapy*
  EDITED BY JESSE H. WRIGHT, M.D., PH.D.

Throughout the country, media coverage is responding to in-creased popular demand for information about the brain—what it does, how it works, and what to expect of it throughout the life cycle. For example, in a special issue of *Scientific American* called "Better Brains: How Neuroscience Will Enhance You," in September 2003, leading researchers summarized exciting new frontiers in psychiatry, including neuroplasticity, new diagnostic technology, new drug development informed by knowledge about gene sequences and molecular configurations, new directions in stress management guided by increased understanding of the effects of stress on the brain, and brain stimulation techniques related to the revolutionary recognition that neurogenesis can occur in the adult brain. This special issue illustrates the enormous excitement about developments in brain science.

In our scientific journals, there is an explosion of information about neuroscience and about the bidirectional nature of brain and behavior. The matter was previously debated as if one had to choose between two camps (mind versus brain), but a rapidly developing new paradigm is replacing this former dichotomy—that the brain influences behavior, and that the mind (ideas, emotions, hopes, aspirations, anxieties, fears, and the wide realm of real and perceived environmental experience) influences the brain. The term *neuropsychiatry* has served as successor to the former term *organic psychiatry* and is contrasted with notions of psychodynamics, such as the concept of unconsciously motivated behavior. As our field evolves and matures, we are developing a new language for meaningful but imperfectly understood earlier concepts. *Subliminal cues* and *indirect memory* are among the terms of our new language, but the emerging understanding that experience itself can activate genes and stimulate protein synthesis, cellular growth, and neurogenesis is a groundbreaking new synthesis of concepts that previously seemed incompatible. Among the remarkable conclusions that these new findings suggest is that psychotherapy can be construed as a biological treatment, in the sense that it has the potential to alter the cellular microanatomy of the brain.

In the context of this rapidly changing scientific and clinical landscape, we selected for the 2004 Review of Psychiatry four broad areas of attention: 1) research findings in developmental psychobiology, 2) current recommendations for neuropsychiatric assessment of patients, 3) new treatments in the form of brain stimulation techniques, and 4) the application of cognitive-behavior therapy as a component of treatment of patients with severely disabling psychiatric disorders.

Perhaps the logical starting place in the 2004 series is *Developmental Psychobiology*, edited by B.J. Casey. Derived from research that uses animal models and studies of early human development, this work summarizes the profound impact of early environmental events. Following a comprehensive overview of the field by Casey, elegant studies of the developmental psychobiology of attachment are presented by Hofer, one of the pioneers in this work. Specific areas of research are then described in detail: the developmental neurobiology of an early maturational task called face processing (Scott and Nelson); findings in the developmental psychobiology of reading disability (McCandliss and Wolmetz); current thinking about the central relevance of early development in the disabling condition Gilles de la Tourette's syndrome (Gallardo, Swain, and Leckman); and the early development of the prefrontal cortex and the implications of these findings in adult-onset schizophrenia (Erickson and Lewis).

Stuart C. Yudofsky and H. Florence Kim, the editors of *Neuropsychiatric Assessment,* have gathered together experts to bring us up to date on the current practice of neuropsychiatric physical diagnosis (Ovsiew); the importance of the neuropsychological examination of psychiatric patients (Getz and Lovell); and the use of electrophysiological testing (Boutros and Struve) and neuropsychiatric laboratory testing (Kim and Yudofsky) in clinical practice. Any focus on neuropsychiatry today must include information about developments in brain imaging; here the clinical usefulness of selected neuroimaging techniques for specific psychiatric disorders is reviewed by Nordahl and Salo.

A particularly interesting area of clinical research, and one with promising potential to provide new treatment techniques, is that of stimulating the brain. The long-known phenomenon of "magnetism" has emerged in a fascinating new incarnation, referred to in its central nervous system applications as transcranial magnetic stimulation (TMS). Sarah H. Lisanby edited *Brain Stimulation in Psychiatric Treatment,* in which TMS is described in connection with its possible use in depression (Schlaepfer and Kosel) and in schizophrenia and other disorders (Hoffman). New applications in psychiatry of deep brain stimulation, a technique showing great promise in Parkinson's disease and other neurological conditions, are reviewed (Greenberg), and the current state of knowledge about magnetic seizure therapy (Lisanby) and vagal nerve stimulation (Sackeim) is presented. All of these roads of investigation have the potential to lead to new, perhaps more effective treatments for our patients.

Finally, in *Cognitive-Behavior Therapy,* edited by Jesse H. Wright, the broadening scope of cognitive therapy is considered with regard to schizophrenia (Scott, Kingdon, and Turkington), bipolar disorder (Basco, McDonald, Merlock, and Rush), medical patients (Sensky), and children and adolescents (Albano, Krain, Podniesinksi, and Ditkowsky). Technological advances in the form of computer-assisted cognitive behavior therapy are presented as well (Wright).

All in all, in our view the selected topics for 2004 represent a rich sampling of the amazing developments taking place in brain science and psychiatric evaluation and treatment. We believe that we have put together an equally relevant menu for 2005, when the Review of Psychiatry Series will include volumes on psychiatric genetics (Kenneth Kendler, editor); sleep disorders and psychiatry (Daniel Buysse, editor); pregnancy and postpartum depression (Lee Cohen, editor); and bipolar disorder (Terence Ketter, Charles Bowden, and Joseph Calabrese, editors).

Introduction

Sarah H. Lisanby, M.D.

The past two decades have seen rapid growth in new and progressively less invasive ways to stimulate the brain for the study and treatment of psychiatric disorders. It is now possible to affect selectively higher cognitive processes and mood systems by stimulating focal regions of the cortex and subcortical structures, directly or indirectly, with electrical currents. But it is important to remember that electricity is not new to psychiatry. Indeed, electroconvulsive therapy (ECT) remains the most effective treatment currently available for severe depression. This year marks the 70th anniversary of the introduction of convulsive therapy. It is an ideal time to examine where the field of brain stimulation in psychiatry is headed over the coming decades.

Novel means of electrically stimulating the central nervous system reviewed in this volume include transcranial magnetic stimulation (TMS), deep brain stimulation (DBS), magnetic seizure therapy (MST), and vagus nerve stimulation (VNS). Although they differ in means of application and degree of invasiveness, all of these procedures are essentially electrical in nature.

In TMS, rapidly alternating magnetic fields are applied to the scalp to induce small electrical currents in the superficial cortex. Administered at moderate intensities, the strength of the induced electrical current is sufficient to depolarize neurons at the site of stimulation and to exert transsynaptic effects at connected regions. At higher intensities, the degree of stimulation can be sufficient to induce a seizure. This higher-dosage convulsive form of magnetic stimulation is called *magnetic seizure therapy* (MST). Both TMS and MST induce far less electricity in the brain than ECT. In addition, TMS and MST are able to stimulate more focal regions of the cortex than is possible with ECT, because magnetic fields pass through tissue without the impedance encountered by direct application of electricity. It is thought that the ability to focus the electrical field induced in the brain will result in fewer side effects than occur with ECT. In addition, the ability to stimulate the brain without inducing a seizure (in the case of TMS) or to induce focal seizures (in the case of MST) is expected to avoid the cognitive side effects caused by the generalized seizures induced by ECT. Results to date support the hypothesis that TMS and MST have fewer cognitive side effects than ECT. At issue is the degree of effectiveness in treating psychiatric disorders. That issue is under active study in a growing number of centers throughout the world.

In the case of TMS, the goal is to determine whether electrical stimulation of neurons alone is sufficient to exert antidepressant effects in the absence of a seizure. If subconvulsive levels of ECT have been shown in controlled trials to be ineffective, why would subconvulsive levels of TMS be any more successful? The answer may lie in the differences between direct application of electricity through the scalp and indirect induction of electricity in the brain by means of a magnetic field. TMS can induce electricity in focal regions of the cortex because magnetic fields pass though tissue unimpeded. The electrical stimulus delivered by ECT is substantially degraded by tissue impedance, and spatial targeting is compromised. Thus subconvulsive levels of ECT are very different in nature from TMS.

The availability of more focal means of brain stimulation challenges workers in our field to identify the specific circuitry that must be modulated for exertion of therapeutic effects. At the same time, we have a method for systematically testing that circuitry. For example, TMS administered to regions of the brain that demonstrate abnormal hyperactivity during hallucinations has been reported to reduce the frequency of auditory hallucinations. That sort of regional specificity is an ideal illustration of the power of using functional neuroimaging to target the intervention. Applying the same approach in treatment of depression has been a bit more complex. For example, it is not known whether cortical or subcortical effects are essential to the antidepressant action of ECT. TMS and MST are essentially cortical interventions, with substantially less impact than ECT on subcortical structures. If these cortical interventions were found to be effective, that would challenge the diencephalic hypothesis of antidepressant action of ECT. Although it is more invasive than the other modalities, DBS has the advantage of being able to reach deeper structures in a highly focal manner. This quality may turn out to be important for illnesses such as obsessive-compulsive disorder, which have a circuitry heavily reliant on subcortical structures. The availability of both cortical interventions and deep brain interventions makes it possible to examine systematically which aspects of the network are essential for therapeutic response in each disorder.

Vagus nerve stimulation consists of an electrical stimulator implanted in the subcutaneous tissue of the chest that administers pulsed electrical stimulation to the vagus nerve in the neck. This device stimulates vagal afferents and activates brainstem nuclei that innervate widespread cortical and subcortical structures. Although VNS is less invasive than DBS, it is more invasive than MST. VNS shares with the other forms of brain stimulation challenges in determining the optimal parameters of stimulation (frequency, amplitude, train duration, pulse width) and in designing adequately masked clinical trials with plausible sham conditions. Unlike the other forms of brain stimulation, VNS is bound by the anatomy of the vagus nerve. Although the operator is at liberty to move the TMS coil or implant the DBS electrode in a desired location of relevance for the illness in question, the effects of VNS are limited to the neuroanatomical connectivity of the vagus nerve. Substantial overlap between the distribution of vagal afferents and circuits critical for antidepressant action would be a distinct advantage. However, there are clear anatomical limits, making it less possible to tailor administration of VNS as easily as the other forms of brain stimulation.

Although none of these technologies is currently approved by the U.S. Food and Drug Administration for treatment of psychiatric disorders, that status may change in the near future. In the meantime, it is important to recognize that wide-scale "off-label" use of these investigational procedures is not recommended. It is imperative that members of the field be able to generate the large multicenter randomized controlled trials needed to demonstrate the efficacy and safety of these procedures. Such studies are under way, and the results expected to come in the next 5 to 10 years will be critical in determining whether and where these interventions fit into our treatment algorithms. Regardless of the ultimate clinical role, is it already clear that these modalities can yield important information regarding the pathophysiological mechanisms of psychiatric disorders that will be of use in developing newer and even more targeted treatments for our patients.

What do these developments in brain stimulation mean for the future of ECT? It is my view that the development of other forms of brain stimulation can only enrich our knowledge about how ECT exerts its profound antidepressant effects. Such knowledge can guide refinements in ECT technique to improve its already excellent risk/benefit ratio. The availability of more brain interventions for treating psychiatric disorders means more choices and a larger range of therapeutic strategies for patients who have conditions that are resistant to conventional treatments. That would clearly be good news for the field and for our patients.

Chapter 1

Transcranial Magnetic Stimulation in Depression

Thomas E. Schlaepfer, M.D.
Markus Kosel, M.D., Ph.D.

Transcranial magnetic stimulation (TMS) is a relatively noninvasive technique used to interfere with the function of small cortical areas through currents induced by alternating magnetic fields emanating from a handheld coil placed directly above the targeted area. This technique has clear effects on a range of measures of brain function and has become an important research tool in neuropsychiatry. TMS has been studied in psychiatry mainly for assessment of its putative therapeutic effects in treatment of refractory major depression. Results of most studies indicate that both low-frequency TMS and higher-frequency (20 Hz) repetitive TMS (rTMS) may have antidepressant properties. These findings are most interesting and open a new avenue of minimally invasive techniques for stimulating the brain in major depression. However, definite therapeutic effects of clinical significance remain to be demonstrated.

Transcranial Magnetic Stimulation— Its Principle of Action

Transcranial magnetic stimulation refers to an in vivo technique of delivering magnetic pulses to the cortex with a handheld stimulating coil, which is applied directly to the head. The equipment

Work reported on in this chapter was supported by grants 4038-044046 and 3231-044523 from the Swiss National Science Foundation to Dr. Schlaepfer.

necessary for delivering TMS consists of two parts: a stimulator, which generates brief pulses of strong electrical currents whose frequency and intensity can be varied, and a stimulation coil connected to the stimulator. The magnetic field generated at the coil passes unimpeded through scalp and skull, inducing an electrical current in the underlying tissue that depolarizes neurons. The main advantages of this method of stimulation are noninvasiveness and the capability of stimulating very small brain volumes. Single, paired, or repetitive magnetic pulses can be generated and delivered. Cortical excitability can be increased or decreased depending on stimulation frequency (Hallett 2000), and TMS has been shown to modify regional cerebral blood flow (Bohning et al. 2000; Catafau et al. 2001).

Transcranial Magnetic Stimulation— Its History

With the observation by Faraday in 1831 that a time-varying magnetic field can induce a current in a nearby conductor, the theoretical basis of inducing depolarizing currents by electromagnetic coils was established. The French scientist d'Arsonval in 1896 reported on the first application of TMS in humans. d'Arsonval induced phosphenes (a flickering-light sensation not elicited by visual perception), vertigo, and syncope in subjects whose heads were placed in a large electromagnetic coil (Geddes 1991). In 1959, Kolin demonstrated for the first time that an alternating magnetic field can stimulate the sciatic nerve of a frog and induce contractions of the gastrocnemius muscle (Geddes 1991). In 1965, Bickford induced muscle twitching in humans by applying a pulsed magnetic field with a maximum field strength of 20,000 to 30,000 gauss to ulnar, peroneal, and sciatic nerves (Geddes 1991). Induction of muscle potentials by magnetic stimulation of the central nervous system was first demonstrated by Barker et al. in 1985. These investigators induced muscle twitching with a coil of 10-cm diameter placed on the scalp over the motor cortex. A brief pulse of 110 microseconds with a peak current of 4,000 amperes was applied, and pulses were delivered at a maximal rate of 0.33 Hz.

With the possibility of noninvasive stimulation of the motor cortex (Figure 1–1), TMS replaced high-voltage transcutaneous electrical stimulation, which had been used in clinical studies mainly for measurement of central motor conduction time. This variable can be altered by a variety of neurological disorders, such as multiple sclerosis, amyotrophic lateral sclerosis, cervical myelopathy, and degenerative ataxic disorders. It seems that TMS has great potential in the intraoperative monitoring of the integrity of motor tracts during surgery on the brain and spinal tract (Murray 1991). TMS has found diagnostic use in neurology for disorders such as demyelinating diseases involving excitability and the connections between the motor cortex and other parts of the nervous system involved in motor pathways (Ziemann and Hallett 2000).

In 1987 Bickford extended the field of TMS research into neuropsychiatry. He was the first to describe transient mood elevation in several healthy volunteers who received single-pulse stimulations to the motor cortex (Bickford et al. 1987). This was the starting point of the scientific investigation of effects of depolarizing magnetic fields in a variety of neuropsychiatric disorders. Soon after, open studies of the effects of TMS on patients with major depression were conducted with single-pulse stimulation at frequencies less than 0.3 Hz (Grisaru et al. 1994; Höflich et al. 1993; Kolbinger et al. 1995). In these studies relatively large areas under the vertex were stimulated bilaterally, and only very few subjects were involved. More recent work has suggested that both slow and fast rTMS may have some value in the treatment of depression.

Effects at Cellular and Systemic Levels

Immediate early gene expression is a useful marker for activation and has been widely used successfully in psychopharmacology. Using this technique, Ji et al. (1998) found that a single train of rTMS applied to rats in vivo induced c-*fos* and c-*jun* expression in different brain regions, including key regions controlling circadian biological rhythms, such as the retina, the paraventricular nucleus of the thalamus, the suprachiasmatic nucleus, and the pi-

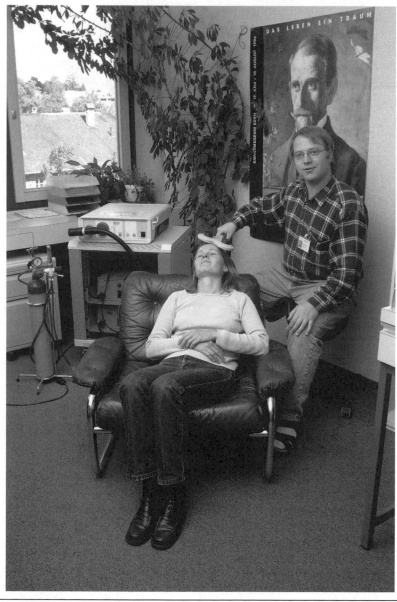

Figure 1–1. Application of repetitive transcranial magnetic stimulation (rTMS).

Depicted is a typical setting for nonconvulsive rTMS studies. The patient is awake, sitting relaxed in a chair while stimulation is applied, here to the left dorsolateral prefrontal cortex. A typical stimulator (here with four booster modules) affording high-frequency stimulation is used. The nearby oxygen tank would be used as the most important therapy in the event of a seizure.

neal gland. The same stimulation parameters earlier were shown to be efficacious in an animal model of depression (Fleischmann et al. 1995). These findings may point to a possible antidepressant mode of action of TMS effects that works by means of circadian rhythms. The finding that immediate to early gene expression is influenced by TMS was replicated and further examined both in vivo and in vitro (Doi et al. 2001; Hausmann et al. 2001).

Keck et al. (2000) used intracerebral microdialysis to measure modulatory effects of frontal rTMS on rat brain in vivo. Up to 50% continuous reduction in arginine vasopressin release occurred within the hypothalamic paraventricular nucleus. In contrast, release of taurine, aspartate, and serine was selectively stimulated within this nucleus. In the dorsal hippocampus the extracellular concentration of dopamine was elevated in response to rTMS. Keck et al. (2000), using intracerebral microdialysis in rats, assessed the effects of rTMS at 20 Hz on the hippocampal, accumbal, and striatal release patterns of dopamine and its metabolites. These investigators found that rTMS of frontal brain regions has a modulatory effect on both mesolimbic and mesostriatal dopaminergic systems and concluded that this effect may contribute to the beneficial effects of rTMS in the treatment of affective disorders (Keck et al. 2002). Using positron emission tomography to examine eight volunteers, Strafellea et al. (2001) found a reduction in raclopride C 11 binding to dopamine receptors in the left dorsal caudate nucleus after left dorsolateral prefrontal cortex (DLPFC) rTMS. This finding implied that rTMS can trigger dopamine release in these brain structures.

Several studies documented the effect of rTMS on plasma levels of a variety of hormones, including cortisol, prolactin, and thyroid-stimulating hormone. Results of these studies were inconclusive, but they indicated that TMS may affect neuroendocrine function (Cohrs et al. 1998; George et al. 1996; Szuba et al. 2001). Depending on the region stimulated, TMS can transiently disrupt or induce activity in focal brain regions. Applied to the visual cortex, for example, strong TMS can produce phosphenes, and stimuli of lower intensity induce transient scotomas (Hallett 2000). Moreover, other functions, such as linguistic processing, can be investigated with rTMS (Flitman et al. 1998). A neuromodulatory effect of subthreshold high-frequency rTMS was observed in 10 subjects. After 1,250 stimulations at 90% motor threshold, intracortical inhibition was measured that persisted at least 10 minutes after rTMS stimulation (Peinemann et al. 2000).

The combination of noninvasive stimulation of the brain coupled with functional neuroimaging techniques offers novel opportunities for investigation of human brain function. It also allows visualization of the effects of TMS, including those distant from the site of stimulation (Bohning et al. 1997, 2000; Paus et al. 1997). For example, in a crossover, randomized study, 10 medication-free subjects with major depression (eight cases unipolar; two, bipolar) received rTMS at the left prefrontal cortex at 100% motor threshold at either 20 Hz or 1 Hz. After 20-Hz treatment, an increase in regional cerebral blood flow was observed in the prefrontal cortex (left greater than right), cingulate gyrus (left much greater than right), left amygdala, bilateral insula, basal ganglia, hippocampus, parahippocampus, thalamus, and cerebellum. After 1-Hz treatment, decreases in regional cerebral blood flow were found only in right prefrontal cortex, left medial cortex, left basal ganglia, and left amygdala. Patients who improved clinically with 1-Hz rTMS tended to worsen with 20-Hz rTMS, and vice versa (Speer et al. 2000).

These multidisciplinary results suggested that TMS has prominent and reproducible effects on the brain. One problem shared with antidepressants is that the link between changes at the cellular level and complex behavioral changes, such as the ones observed in depression, has been difficult to establish. The field of neuropsychiatric research in TMS has suffered somewhat from a top-down approach in which early promising results in the study of depression led to enthusiasm for clinical studies without sufficient basic data on neurobiological factors. Approaches integrating findings from all levels of brain systems— molecular to behavioral—are extremely important and should be undertaken to support ongoing clinical research.

The magnetic field induced by TMS interacts with an extremely complex biological system in which essential interactions between brain and mind take place (Kandel 1998, 1999). The impact of these fields on brain systems is difficult to evaluate, because monitoring of functions of the living human brain is possible only by assessment of summation responses determined by the action of tens of thousands or more cells. The current models of psychiatric disorders encompass functional systems at molecular, cellular, neurotransmitter, organ, systemic, or individual and social levels that are not well understood. Presenting the mechanisms of action of TMS as either a research or a treatment tool challenges old hypotheses of brain function and allows generation of new hypotheses. Several acute and chronic alterations at different levels, ranging from changes in gene expression of cells in the central nervous system to alterations in mood and behavior, have been documented during and after application of TMS.

Side Effects

Compared with other methods of brain stimulation, rTMS can be considered relatively safe because it is noninvasive. Of major concern are involuntarily induced seizure, local pain during application, changes in auditory performance due to the noise generated in the coil by the passing electrical current, headache, and potential alterations in cognitive function. Until now, mainly short-term problems (application of TMS, follow-up period of a few weeks) were addressed in research applications. Long-term concerns also must be addressed. These concerns include long-lasting cognitive impairment, sleep problems, and problems linked to the manner in which strong magnetic fields affect the brain.

Immediate and Short-Term Risks

Seizures

The risk of causing a seizure is the primary safety concern with TMS. Even if this risk is primarily associated with rTMS, single-pulse stimulation has been reported to produce seizures in patients with large cerebral infarcts, contusions, or other structural brain lesions. According to Wassermann (2000), seizures do not occur in patients with completely subcortical lesions. According to the same author, a few articles describe induction of seizures in epilepsy patients without gross lesions. In at least 6 volunteers without depression and at least 2 patients with depression, unplanned seizure occurred during rTMS stimulation (Wassermann 2000). None of the subjects who had rTMS-induced seizures experienced lasting sequelae. Electroencephalographic recordings became normal after at least 2 days. Recorded effects were mild recall deficits, which returned to normal after 24 hours, in two individuals and significant anxiety concerning the possibility of a recurrent seizure in one subject. At the time of this writing, several thousand individuals had undergone rTMS treatments. It seems reasonable to assume that under conditions conforming to established safety guidelines, development of seizure activity is extremely unlikely (Wassermann 1998).

Cognitive Impairment

Observations concerning cognitive function after TMS administration are mainly short-term. Depending on the site of stimulation, rTMS can produce transient disruption of various cerebral functions. Observations include a significant decrease in score on a memory subtest within an hour after stimulation with 150 trains of rTMS at 15 Hz and 120% motor threshold delivered at four different positions (Flitman et al. 1998). Reviewing these results, Lorberbaum and Wasserman (2000) concluded these cognitive effects were due to subconvulsive epileptic activity or that the threshold for adverse effects on memory might be near that of seizure. Loo et al. (2001) reported results from a study in which 12 subjects with major depression received rTMS for 4 weeks. After 4 weeks no significant changes in neuropsychological functioning were observed. In a study with 15 patients with major depression who received left dorsolateral rTMS, Shajahan et al. (2002) found that cortical excitability and functional connectivity were influenced, but no deterioration in neuropsychological function was observed. Another group of investigators (Moser et al. 2002) found that patients receiving rTMS had significantly improved scores on the Trail Making Test B, a test of cognitive flexibility and conceptual tracking.

Cardiovascular Effects

No significant changes in blood pressure and heart rate during or after administration of rTMS have been reported (Foerster et al. 1997).

Auditory Function

No significant changes in auditory threshold were observed in a study involving 12 depressed subjects undergoing rTMS for 4 weeks when they were observed for 4 weeks after the end of the study (Loo et al. 2001).

Headache

Application of TMS can cause local pain resulting from direct stimulation of muscles under the coil and from stimulation of facial and scalp nerves. The procedure is generally more painful at higher intensities and frequencies. Approximately 5% to 20% of subjects experience tension headache after rTMS sessions (George et al. 1999).

Long-Term Risks

It is important to carefully consider whether application of rTMS can cause brain damage in the broadest sense. Potential mechanisms for damage theoretically include heating of neuronal tissue, excitotoxicity, and influences of magnetic fields. The amount of current induced in the brain by rTMS is substantially lower than that induced by electroconvulsive therapy (ECT), and both rTMS and ECT are orders of magnitude below levels that would cause appreciable tissue heating or neuronal damage. Results of animal studies show no evidence of neuronal damage attributable to rTMS.

The kind of low-frequency, high-strength magnetic fields delivered to the human brain during rTMS are not known in other applications. Considerable evidence has accumulated about constant, strong static magnetic fields with the introduction of magnetic resonance imaging techniques in medicine. These fields have approximately the same strength as those produced by rTMS, and the duration of exposure is much longer. Since the introduction of magnetic resonance imaging, more than 150 million examinations have been performed, and only seven deaths have been attributed to these procedures (Schenck 2000). One death involved a ferromagnetic cerebral aneurysm clip, and five occurred during examinations of patients with cardiac pacemakers. High-frequency (approximately 1,000 MHz) electromagnetic fields, as generated by cell phones, have been investigated with regard to adverse health effects, and no adverse effects have been found. Interestingly enough, fields generated at those frequencies have been demonstrated to induce changes in sleep electroencephalographic patterns 20 to 50 minutes after electromagnetic waves were applied to awake subjects (Huber et al. 2000). In rTMS, very different energies and frequencies of electromagnetic fields are applied to the human brain. In a safety study, rTMS at therapeutic parameters has been demonstrated to have no significant effects on sleep EEG (Graf et al. 2001).

Effects on Mood of Healthy Volunteers

It is important to elucidate the exact structural and functional bases of affect to understand the neurobiological mechanisms of, and putative therapeutic interventions for, human disorders such as depression and mania. Converging evidence from different areas of research supports the hypothesis that mood is regulated by an interconnected network of brain regions encompassing prefrontal, cingulate, parietal, and temporal cortical regions as well as parts of the striatum, thalamus, and hypothalamus. Among these, the limbic system integrates external stimuli with internal drives and is part of a distributed neural network that marks stimuli and events with positive or negative value (Aggleton 1993). Lesions of this network from tumor, infarction, or transient disruption often result in mood changes. In addition, alterations of cerebral blood flow and metabolism in the dorsolateral, ventrolateral, orbitofrontal, and medial frontal regions as well as the subgenual prefrontal and anterior cingulate cortex have been demonstrated in patients with major depression (Mayberg 1997; Soares and Mann 1997). Some researchers have concluded that the prefrontal cortex is implicated in mood generation and modulation, but this view is not universal (George et al. 1995a; Lane et al. 1997; Paradiso et al. 1997).

rTMS has been used in healthy subjects to help elucidate the basic neurophysiological mechanisms of mood generation and modulation by stimulating the DLPFC. The effect of prefrontal rTMS on mood systems of healthy volunteers was investigated in six studies. In three of the studies, rTMS over the left prefrontal cortex transiently induced a decrease in self-rated happiness and an increase in sadness compared with the effects of right prefrontal cortical rTMS (Dearing et al. 1997; George et al. 1996; Pascual-Leone et al. 1996). The three more recent studies (Cohrs et al. 1998; Mosimann et al. 2000; Nedjat et al. 1998) showed no effects on mood in healthy volunteers.

Effects on Mood in Major Depression

Because of its ability to focally interfere with neuronal circuits, rTMS has been proposed and subsequently researched as a putative therapeutic approach to the treatment of refractory major depression (Nemeroff 1996; Nestler 1998). As in studies of mood modulation by rTMS, the DLPFC has been the most important target for stimulation in studies of major depression. George et al. (1995b) reported the results of the first open study of the effects of rTMS. The subjects were six patients with refractory depression treated with five daily rTMS sessions to the left DLPFC. The investigators found that two patients in the study experienced improvement evidenced by a reduction of 26% in Hamilton Rating Scale for Depression (Ham-D) score. Open and masked studies of rTMS to the left DLPFC followed with varying results. Results of a relatively large open study showed that 21 (42%) of 50 patients responded to five daily rTMS sessions, elderly patients exhibiting a considerably lower response rate (Figiel et al. 1998). In another open trial, a 2-week treatment study resulted in a 41% decrease in Ham-D score (Triggs et al. 1999). However, other open studies demonstrated no antidepressant activity of rTMS (Schouten et al. 1999).

In sham-controlled, single-masked studies of rTMS for treatment-resistant depression, effect sizes varied considerably. In a within-subject crossover, sham-controlled study with 12 depressed patients treated for 2 weeks with stimulation of the left DLPFC, only somewhat modest antidepressant efficacy of rTMS was found (George et al. 1997). In a more recent study, an antidepressant effect occurred in 20 subjects. This effect was statistically different from the effect of sham stimulation when similar stimulation parameters were used in a parallel design, but still only modest clinical effect occurred (Berman et al. 2000). In some studies a low stimulation intensity of 80% of motor threshold was used. In general, it seems that higher intensity may be more effective, although Loo et al. (1999) found no differences between active and sham rTMS when they used a much higher stimulation intensity (110% of motor threshold). This observation was confirmed in a relatively older outpatient patient group (Mosimann et al., in press). In a large sham-controlled trial with 71 patients in which low-frequency rTMS was used, the investigators found that 1-Hz stimulation of the *right* DLPFC was significantly more effective than sham stimulation (Klein et al. 1999). It is unclear whether stimulation of the *left* DLPFC at these parameters would have had the same effect. The effect of frequency was compared in a study in which 18 patients were randomized to single-pulse TMS, 10-Hz rTMS, and sham rTMS delivered to the left DLPFC. A mild antidepressant effect with single-pulse TMS was demonstrated (Padberg et al. 1999). In a sham-controlled trial in which 20 patients were randomly assigned to receive an equivalent number of pulses at 5 Hz or 20 Hz over 2 weeks, both active groups experienced 45% reduction in depression severity ratings, and none of the patients responded to sham stimulation (George et al. 2000). This finding suggests that lower frequencies may have therapeutic efficacy, which is important because slow rTMS is associated with lower seizure risk. Results of an analysis of treatment response and cerebral metabolism suggested that patients with hypometabolism at baseline may respond better to high-frequency stimulation (20 Hz), whereas those with baseline hypermetabolism responded better to 1-Hz stimulation (Kimbrell et al. 1999). However, the effects of rTMS on mood examined in this study were not statistically significant.

There are indications that TMS stimulation at higher amplitudes may be more efficacious (Padberg et al. 2002). Mosimann et al. (2002) found a negative correlation between distance from coil to cortex and antidepressant response. This value was expressed as percentage of decrease in Ham-D rating before and after treatment in a relatively older patient group with treatment-refractory major depression. The results showed a process of prefrontal atrophy may outpace motor cortex atrophy in chronically depressed middle-aged subjects. An even more recent study was conducted with 31 patients experiencing a pharmacotherapy-resistant major depressive episode. These patients were randomly assigned to three treatment groups receiving rTMS at different stimulation intensities. Improvement of depressive symptoms after rTMS significantly increased with stimulation intensity across the three groups. This finding supports the hypothesis of a relationship between stimulation intensity of rTMS and antidepressant efficacy (Padberg et al. 2002).

These observations together with the established fact that therapeutic seizures have a strong and reliable effect on depression led to development of another method: rTMS at convulsive levels as a more targeted form of convulsive therapy (see Chapter 4, "Magnetic Seizure Therapy," in this volume). Efficacy and side effects of ECT seem to depend on the path of the current passed through the brain (Sackeim 2000; Sackeim et al. 1993). Therefore targeting seizures to focal cortical areas, such as regions of the prefrontal cortex, may reduce some of the side effects of convulsive treatment. Magnetic seizure therapy has been tested in proof-of-concept studies with both nonhuman primates and patients (Lisanby et al. 2001). Preliminary results on cognitive side effects of the treatment compared with those of ECT have been obtained (Lisanby et al. 2003). Much additional research is needed to evaluate the putative clinical efficacy of this approach and to determine whether it has significant advantages over ECT in terms of similar effects and a better side-effect profile.

Some early data in relatively smaller patient populations in open (Dannon et al. 2002; Grunhaus et al. 2000) and randomized (Janicak et al. 2002) trials suggest that even nonconvulsive rTMS at 110% of motor threshold has efficacy similar to that of ECT in patients with major depression. In the framework of a large meta-analysis of rTMS studies of depression, Burt et al. (2002) conducted an analysis of studies directly comparing rTMS to ECT. The general effect size for TMS in these studies was greater than in the studies comparing TMS to sham—most likely reflecting a subject selection bias. The authors suggested that TMS probably works best in patients who are candidates for ECT, although the possibility of placebo effects cannot be ruled out because the ECT/rTMS comparisons were not double-masked.

The method of meta-analysis has been applied to the body of literature in the field of rTMS in depression (Burt et al. 2002; Holtzheimer et al. 2001; Martin et al. 2002, 2003; McNamara et al. 2001). Although each set of investigators included different studies and applied different methods of analysis, all found that the antidepressant effect of rTMS is higher than that of sham treatment. Overall this antidepressant effect is mild to moderate, and the reviews do not agree in terms of *clinical* significance of the method.

Conclusion

The data on clinical efficacy of rTMS in mood disorders are not unequivocal but nevertheless are interesting and encouraging. Rigorously controlled, double-masked multicenter trials are urgently needed to adequately address the question of the clinical efficacy of rTMS. Before such studies are performed, technical problems in the application of TMS have to be solved; for example, more satisfactory sham conditions must be developed. Analogies to antidepressant drug development must be conducted with valid phase II trials. Crucial unanswered questions remain, including the long-term efficacy of TMS, prevention of relapse, and long-term side effects. The key findings in the immediate treatment of depression have not been systematically replicated, and effect sizes have been small and variable. Sources of variability across studies include differences in stimulation settings, concomitant medications, and different characteristics of patient samples. In addition, simple and economical methods for precise and reproducible coil placement are needed because this factor is likely important for effectiveness (Kozel et al. 2000). In much of this work, the magnitude of antidepressant effect, although often statistically significant, has been below the threshold of clinical usefulness (Berman et al. 2000) and has not lived up to expectations raised by encouraging results in animal studies. Furthermore, the persistence of antidepressant effects beyond the 1- to 2-week treatment period has rarely been examined. Initial evidence suggests that the beneficial effects may be transitory, making the development of maintenance strategies important if rTMS is to become clinically applicable.

Establishing whether nonconvulsive rTMS has antidepressant properties is of theoretical importance because positive data support the notion that focally targeted manipulations of cortical function can result in mood improvement. Nonetheless, the future clinical usefulness of rTMS as an antidepressant therapy is far from certain. In a systematic review of published and unpublished studies on the effectiveness of rTMS in the treatment of refractory major depression, Martin et al. (2003) found both a relative lack in overall quality of studies (compared with drug registration trials) and a lack of main effect.

There is no consensus about the exact mechanisms of action by which rTMS induces antidepressant effects. However, this also is the case for many other antidepressant treatments. Research on rTMS has mainly been empirical. Many variables of rTMS application must be carefully explored to find the most efficacious treatment. This process will most likely be slow, because only public funding is available for such studies. Nevertheless, rTMS has clear effects on the brain that are certainly remarkable. It may be that rTMS is a treatment modality in search of a suitable psychiatric application, which may well be depression at other values of stimulation.

From the viewpoint of neuroscientists, TMS is a method with great potential as a research tool (Hallett 2000; Lisanby et al. 2000, 2002). This technique, by itself and combined with other methods such as electroencephalography and neuroimaging, may be useful for testing functional connectivity, neuroplasticity, information processing (e.g., in the visual system), indirect and direct motor control, and aspects of mood control. It affords testing of general hypotheses of the function of the brain at different levels and hypotheses of the underlying pathologic mechanism of neuropsychiatric disorders. Even if early enthusiasm, which prevailed after early studies of clinical effects in the treatment of mood disorders, has settled down, rTMS will be useful as an investigational tool for basic and clinical research.

References

Aggleton JP: The contribution of the amygdala to normal and abnormal emotional states. Trends Neurosci 16:328–333, 1993

Barker AT, Jalinous R, Freeston IL: Non-invasive magnetic stimulation of human motor cortex. Lancet 2:1106–1107, 1985

Berman RM, Narasimhan M, Sanacora G, et al: A randomized clinical trial of repetitive transcranial magnetic stimulation in the treatment of major depression. Biol Psychiatry 47:332–337, 2000

Bickford RG, Guidi M, Fortesque P, et al: Magnetic stimulation of human peripheral nerve and brain: response enhancement by combined magnetoelectrical technique. Neurosurgery 20:110–116, 1987

Bohning DE, Pecheny AP, Epstein CM, et al: Mapping transcranial magnetic stimulation (TMS) fields in vivo with MRI. Neuroreport 8:2535–2538, 1997

Bohning DE, Shastri A, Wassermann EM, et al: BOLD-fMRI response to single-pulse transcranial magnetic stimulation (TMS). J Magn Reson Imaging 11:569–574, 2000

Burt T, Lisanby SH, Sackeim HA, et al: Neuropsychiatric applications of transcranial magnetic stimulation: a meta analysis. Int J Neuropsychopharmacol 5:73–103, 2002

Catafau A, Perez V, Gironell A, et al: SPECT mapping of cerebral activity changes induced by repetitive transcranial magnetic stimulation in depressed patients: a pilot study. Psychiatry Res 106:151–160, 2001

Cohrs S, Tergau F, Riech S, et al: High-frequency repetitive transcranial magnetic stimulation delays rapid eye movement sleep. Neuroreport 9:3439–3443, 1998

Dannon PN, Dolberg OT, Schreiber S, et al: Three and six-month outcome following courses of either ECT or rTMS in a population of severely depressed individuals: preliminary report. Biol Psychiatry 51:687–690, 2002

Dearing J, George MS, Greenberg BD, et al: Mood effects of prefrontal repetitive high frequency transcranial magnetic stimulation (rTMS) in healthy volunteers. CNS Spectrums 2:53–68, 1997

Doi W, Sato D, Fukuzako H, et al: c-*Fos* expression in rat brain after repetitive transcranial magnetic stimulation. Neuroreport 12:1307–1310, 2001

Figiel GS, Epstein C, McDonald WM, et al: The use of rapid-rate transcranial magnetic stimulation (rTMS) in refractory depressed patients. J Neuropsychiatry Clin Neurosci 10:20–25, 1998

Fleischmann A, Prolov K, Abarbanel J, et al: The effect of transcranial magnetic stimulation of rat brain on behavioral models of depression. Brain Res 698:130–132, 1995

Flitman, S, Grafman J, Wassermann EM, et al: Linguistic processing during repetitive transcranial magnetic stimulation. Neurology 50:175–181, 1998

Foerster A, Schmitz JM, Nouri S, et al: Safety of rapid-rate transcranial magnetic stimulation: heart rate and blood pressure changes. Electroencephalogr Clin Neurophysiol 104:207–212, 1997

Geddes LA: History of magnetic stimulation of the nervous system. J Clin Neurophysiol 8:3–9, 1991

George MS, Ketter TA, Parekh PI, et al: Brain activity during transient sadness and happiness in healthy women. Am J Psychiatry 152:341–351, 1995a

George MS, Wassermann EM, Williams WA, et al: Daily repetitive transcranial magnetic stimulation (rTMS) improves mood in depression. Neuroreport 6:1853–1856, 1995b

George MS, Wassermann EM, Williams WA, et al: Changes in mood and hormone levels after rapid-rate transcranial magnetic stimulation (rTMS) of the prefrontal cortex. J Neuropsychiatry Clin Neurosci 8:172–180, 1996

George MS, Wassermann EM, Kimbrell TA, et al: Mood improvement following daily left prefrontal repetitive transcranial magnetic stimulation in patients with depression: a placebo-controlled crossover trial. Am J Psychiatry 154:1752–1756, 1997

George MS, Lisanby SH, Sackheim HA: Transcranial magnetic stimulation: applications in neuropsychiatry. Arch Gen Psychiatry 56:300–311, 1999

George MS, Nahas Z, Molloy M, et al: A controlled trial of daily left prefrontal cortex TMS for treating depression. Biol Psychiatry 48:962–970, 2000

Graf T, Engeler J, Achermann P, et al: High frequency repetitive transcranial magnetic stimulation (rTMS) of the left dorsolateral cortex: EEG topography during waking and subsequent sleep. Psychiatry Res 107:1–9, 2001

Grisaru N, Yaroslavsky Y, Abarbanel J, et al: Transcranial magnetic stimulation in depression and schizophrenia. Eur Neuropsychopharmacol 4:287–288, 1994

Grunhaus L, Dannon PN, Schreiber S, et al: Repetitive transcranial magnetic stimulation is as effective as electroconvulsive therapy in the treatment of nondelusional major depressive disorder: an open study. Biol Psychiatry 47:314–324, 2000

Hallett M: Transcranial magnetic stimulation and the brain. Nature 406:147–150, 2000

Hausmann A, Marksteiner J, Hinterhuber H, et al: Magnetic stimulation induces neuronal c-fos via tetrodotoxin-sensitive sodium channels in organotypic cortex brain slices in rat. Neurosci Lett 310:105–108, 2001

Höflich G, Kasper S, Hufnagel A, et al: Application of transcranial magnetic stimulation in the treatment of drug-resistant major depression: a report of two cases. Hum Psychopharmacol 8:361–365, 1993

Holtzheimer PE 3rd, Russo J, Avery DH: A meta-analysis of repetitive transcranial magnetic stimulation in the treatment of depression. Psychopharmacol Bull 35:149–169, 2001

Huber R, Graf T, Cote KA, et al: Exposure to pulsed high-frequency electromagnetic field during waking affects human sleep EEG. Neuroreport 11:3321–3325, 2000

Janicak PG, Dowd SM, Martis B, et al: Repetitive transcranial magnetic stimulation versus electroconvulsive therapy for major depression: preliminary results of a randomized trial. Biol Psychiatry 51:659–667, 2002

Ji RR, Schlaepfer TE, Aizenman CD, et al: Repetitive transcranial magnetic stimulation activates specific regions in rat brain. Proc Natl Acad Sci U S A 95: 15635–15640, 1998

Kandel ER: A new intellectual framework for psychiatry. Am J Psychiatry 155: 457–469, 1998

Kandel ER: Biology and the future of psychoanalysis: a new intellectual framework for psychiatry revisited. Am J Psychiatry 156:505–524, 1999

Keck ME, Sillaber I, Ebner K, et al: Acute transcranial magnetic stimulation of frontal brain regions selectively modulates the release of vasopressin, biogenic amines and amino acids in the rat brain. Eur J Neurosci 12:3713–3720, 2000

Keck ME, Welt T, Muller MB, et al: Repetitive transcranial magnetic stimulation increases the release of dopamine in the mesolimbic and mesostriatal system. Neuropharmacology 43:101–109, 2002

Kimbrell TA, Little JT, Dunn RT, et al: Frequency dependence of antidepressant response to left prefrontal repetitive transcranial magnetic stimulation (rTMS) as a function of baseline cerebral glucose metabolism. Biol Psychiatry 46:1603–1613, 1999

Klein E, Kreinin I, Chistyakov A, et al: Therapeutic efficacy of right prefrontal slow repetitive transcranial magnetic stimulation in major depression: a double-blind controlled study. Arch Gen Psychiatry 56:315–320, 1999

Kolbinger HM, Höflich G, Hufnagel A, et al: Transcranial magnetic stimulation (TMS) in the treatment of major depression. Hum Psychopharmacol 10:305–310, 1995

Kozel FA, Nahas Z, deBrux C, et al: How coil-cortex distance relates to age, motor threshold, and antidepressant response to repetitive transcranial magnetic stimulation. J Neuropsychiatry Clin Neurosci 12:376–384, 2000

Lane RD, Reiman EM, Ahern GL, et al: Neuroanatomical correlates of happiness, sadness, and disgust. Am J Psychiatry 154:926–933, 1997

Lisanby SH, Luber B, Perera T, et al: Transcranial magnetic stimulation: application in basic neuroscience and neuropsychopharmacology. Int J Neuropsychopharmacol 3:259–273, 2000

Lisanby SH, Schlaepfer TE, Fisch HU, et al: Magnetic seizure therapy of major depression. Arch Gen Psychiatry 58:303–305, 2001

Lisanby SH, Kinnunen LH, Crupain MJ, et al: Applications of TMS to therapy in psychiatry. J Clin Neurophysiol 18:344–360, 2002

Lisanby SH, Luber B, Schlaepfer TE, et al: Safety and feasibility of magnetic seizure therapy (MST) in major depression: randomized within-subject comparison with electroconvulsive therapy. Neuropsychopharmacology 10:1852–1865, 2003

Loo C, Mitchell P, Sachdev P, et al: Double-blind controlled investigation of transcranial magnetic stimulation for the treatment of resistant major depression. Am J Psychiatry 156:946–948, 1999

Loo C, Sachdev P, Elsayed H, et al: Effects of a 2- to 4-week course of repetitive transcranial magnetic stimulation (rTMS) on neuropsychologic functioning, electroencephalogram, and auditory threshold in depressed patients. Biol Psychiatry 49:615–623, 2001

Lorberbaum JP, Wassermann EM: Safety concerns of TMS, in Transcranial Magnetic Stimulation in Neuropsychiatry. Edited by George MS, Belmaker RH. Washington DC, American Psychiatric Press, 2000, pp 141–161

Martin J, Barbanoj M, Perez V, et al: Transcranial magnetic stimulation for treating depression. Cochrane Database Syst Rev CD003493, 2002

Martin JL, Barbanoj MJ, Schlaepfer TE, et al: Repetitive transcranial magnetic stimulation for the treatment of depression: systematic review and meta-analysis. Br J Psychiatry 182:480–491, 2003

Mayberg HS: Limbic-cortical dysregulation: a proposed model of depression. J Neuropsychiatry Clin Neurosci 8:471–481, 1997

McNamara B, Ray JL, Arthurs OJ, et al: Transcranial magnetic stimulation for depression and other psychiatric disorders. Psychol Med 31:1141–1146, 2001

Moser DJ, Jorge RE, Manes F, et al: Improved executive functioning following repetitive transcranial magnetic stimulation. Neurology 58:1288–1290, 2002

Mosimann UP, Rihs TA, Engeler J, et al: Mood effects of repetitive transcranial stimulation (rTMS) of left prefrontal cortex in healthy volunteers. Psychiatry Res 94:251–256, 2000

Mosimann UP, Marré SC, Werlen S, et al: Antidepressant effects of repetitive transcranial magnetic stimulation in the elderly: correlation between effect size and coil-cortex distance. Arch Gen Psychiatry 58:560–561, 2002

Mosimann UP, Schmitt W, Kosel M, et al: Repetitive transcranial magnetic stimulation (rTMS) as a putative treatment for major depression: a sham-controlled study in relatively older patients. Psychiatry Res (in press)

Murray NM: Magnetic stimulation of cortex: clinical applications. J Clin Neurophysiol 8:66–76, 1991

Nedjat S, Folkerts HW, Michael ND, et al: Evaluation of the side effects after rapid-rate transcranial magnetic stimulation over the left prefrontal cortex in normal volunteers (abstract). Electroencephalogr Clin Neurophysiol 107:96, 1998

Nemeroff CB: Augmentation strategies in patients with refractory depression. Depress Anxiety 4:169–181, 1996

Nestler E: Antidepressant treatments in the 21st century. Biol Psychiatry 44:526–533, 1998

Padberg F, Zwanzger P, Thoma H, et al: Repetitive transcranial magnetic stimulation (rTMS) in pharmacotherapy-refractory major depression: comparative study of fast, slow and sham rTMS. Psychiatry Res 88:163–171, 1999

Padberg F, Zwanzger P, Kekc ME, et al: Repetitive transcranial magnetic stimulation (rTMS) in major depression: relation between efficacy and stimulation intensity. Neuropsychopharmacology 27:638–645, 2002

Paradiso S, Robinson RG, Andreasen NC, et al: Emotional activation of limbic circuitry in elderly normal subjects in a PET study. Am J Psychiatry 154:384–389, 1997

Pascual-Leone A, Catala MD, Pascual-Leone Pascual A, et al: Lateralized effect of rapid-rate transcranial magnetic stimulation of the prefrontal cortex on mood. Neurology 46:499–502, 1996

Paus T, Jech R, Thompson CJ, et al: Transcranial magnetic stimulation during positron emission tomography: a new method for studying connectivity of the human cerebral cortex. J Neurosci 17:3178–3184, 1997

Peinemann A, Lehner C, Mentschel C, et al: Subthreshold 5-Hz repetitive transcranial magnetic stimulation of the human primary motor cortex reduces intracortical paired-pulse inhibition. Neurosci Lett 296:21–24, 2000

Sackeim HA: Repetitive transcranial magnetic stimulation: what are the next steps? Biol Psychiatry 48:959–961, 2000

Sackeim HA, Prudic J, Devanand DP, et al: Effects of stimulus intensity and electrode placement on the efficacy and cognitive effects of electroconvulsive therapy. N Engl J Med 328:839–846, 1993

Schenck JF: Safety of strong, static magnetic fields. J Magn Reson Imaging 12:2–19, 2000

Schouten EA, D'Alfonso AA, Nolen WA, et al: Mood improvement from transcranial magnetic stimulation. Am J Psychiatry 156:669–670, 1999

Shajahan PM, Glabus MF, Steele JD, et al: Left dorso-lateral repetitive transcranial magnetic stimulation affects cortical excitability and functional connectivity, but does not impair cognition in major depression. Prog Neuropsychopharmacol Biol Psychiatry 26:945–954, 2002

Soares JC, Mann JJ: The anatomy of mood disorders: review of structural neuroimaging studies. Biol Psychiatry 41:86–106, 1997

Speer AM, Kimbrell TA, Wassermann EM, et al: Opposite effects of high and low frequency rTMS on regional brain activity in depressed patients. Biol Psychiatry 48:1133–1141, 2000

Strafella AP, Paus T, Barrett J, et al: Repetitive transcranial magnetic stimulation of the human prefrontal cortex induces dopamine release in the caudate nucleus. J Neurosci 21:RC157, 2001

Szuba MP, O'Reardon JP, Rai AS, et al: Acute mood and thyroid stimulating hormone effects of transcranial magnetic stimulation in major depression. Biol Psychiatry 50:22–27, 2001

Triggs WJ, McCoy KJ, Greer R, et al: Effects of left frontal transcranial magnetic simulation on depressed mood, cognition, and corticomotor threshold. Biol Psychiatry 45:1440–1445, 1999

Wassermann EM: Risk and safety of repetitive transcranial magnetic stimulation: report and suggested guidelines for the International Workshop on the Safety of Repetitive Transcranial Magnetic Stimulation, June 5–7, 1996. Electroencephalogr Clin Neurophysiol 108:1–16, 1998

Wassermann EM: Side effects of repetitive transcranial magnetic stimulation. Depress Anxiety 12:124–129, 2000

Ziemann U, Hallett M: Basic neurophysiological studies with TMS, in Transcranial Magnetic Stimulation in Neuropsychiatry. Edited by George MS, Belmaker RH. Washington DC, American Psychiatric Press, 2000, pp 45–98

Chapter 2

Transcranial Magnetic Stimulation Studies of Schizophrenia and Other Disorders

Ralph E. Hoffman, M.D.

Transcranial magnetic stimulation (TMS) is a new tool for probing and altering function of selected areas of the brain. In this chapter, I review studies of repetitive TMS (rTMS) in patients with schizophrenia and other disorders that may have treatment implications. rTMS studies of major depression are considered in Chapter 1 of this volume.

rTMS studies can be divided into two types, the first conducted with stimulation at higher frequency ranges (i.e., ≥5 times per second, or ≥5 Hz) and the second examining effects of lower frequency (i.e., once per second, or 1 Hz) stimulation. Post et al. (1997) observed that these rTMS stimulation parameters parallel those used in animal studies of neuroplasticity in which electrical stimulation was used. Higher-frequency direct electrical stimulation of neural tissue can produce *long-term potentiation* (LTP) of transsynaptic signal propagation as well as kindling of seizure

Studies of auditory hallucinations have been supported by a National Alliance for Research on Schizophrenia and Depression Independent Investigator Award, a Donaghue Community and Clinical Issues Award, National Institute of Mental Health grants R21 MH63326 and R01 MH50557, the Chrysalis Fund, National Institutes of Health/National Center for Research Resources/General Clinical Research Center program grant RR00125, and the Department of Mental Health and Addiction Services of the State of Connecticut.

phenomena. In contrast, low-frequency, direct electrical stimulation curtails synaptic transmission, an effect referred to as *long-term depression* (LTD). The Post group proposed that brain stimulation obtained with pulsed magnetic fields administered at the scalp level produces effects paralleling those of LTP and LTD administered at the same frequency.

This conceptual framework is consistent with that for studies of rTMS in human subjects in which cortical reactivity was considered. In the 5–20 Hz frequency range, rTMS delivered to motor cortex appears to facilitate cortical responses (Pascual-Leone et al. 1994) as measured with electromyographic recordings of the peripheral musculature. A more recent study using oxygen-15 positron emission tomography (PET) had parallel findings after a series of 10 treatments with 20-Hz rTMS. rTMS was delivered to the left prefrontal cortex in patients with depression (Speer et al. 2000). Repeated scanning 72 hours after the TMS protocol revealed increases in regional cerebral blood flow in the prefrontal cortex, as well as the cingulate gyrus and amygdala. These data suggested that multiple exposures of high-frequency rTMS to one area have activating effects that are propagated to other functionally linked brain areas.

One-hertz rTMS delivered to the motor cortex produces the opposite effect, namely reduction of cortical responses (Chen et al. 1997). As in the case of higher-frequency rTMS, suppressive effects of 1-Hz rTMS can be propagated to other regions not directly stimulated. For example, 1-Hz rTMS of left motor cortex reduces motor evoked potentials elicited by single-pulse TMS to the right motor cortex (Wassermann et al. 1998), an effect presumably mediated by transcallosal projections. Moreover, 1-Hz rTMS to motor cortex was found to diminish the *Bereitschaftspotential* (Rossi et al. 2000), a slow negative potential preceding motor actions that arises in the supplementary motor area of the frontal cortex. Supplementary motor area also exchanges extensive projections with the motor cortex. Effects of 1-Hz rTMS have been explored in nonmotor cortical areas. Visual cortex excitability can be assessed by determination of the threshold for inducing visual phosphenes by single-pulse TMS to the visual cortex (Boroojerdi et al. 2000). A 15-minute pulse train of 1-Hz rTMS to this region was observed to increase phosphene thresholds, indicating decreased cortex excitability. Speer et al. (2000) used oxygen-15 PET to study effects of 1-Hz rTMS delivered to the left prefrontal cortex of depressed patients. Reductions in prefrontal blood flow were detected after rTMS, albeit on the right side rather than the stimulated, left side. Blood flow activation in the left amygdala also reduced, a finding that suggested multiple exposures of 1-Hz rTMS have effects that propagate to other functionally connected regions.

The results of these studies provided the conceptual basis for studies of rTMS in a range of clinical disorders.

Motor Disorders

The abundant literature demonstrating suppressive effects of 1-Hz rTMS delivered to motor cortex (see Hoffman and Cavus 2002 for review) has produced an interest in using similar protocols in clinical populations with motoric abnormalities.

Wedegaertner et al. (1997) studied effects of 1-Hz rTMS on action myoclonus. rTMS was administered for 30 minutes daily. Two of the patients received stimulation for 5 days, and one patient received stimulation for 3 days. Two patients also received single-masked sham stimulation before the active trial. Amplitude of action myoclonus was reduced 33% for active stimulation, but no effects were detected for sham stimulation. Duration of effects was approximately 2 hours after each rTMS session.

Another application of low-frequency rTMS has been in writer's cramp, which is characterized by excessive muscular activation during writing. In some cases, when handwriting impairment is accompanied by impairment of other motor skills, this condition is considered a focal dystonia. TMS is a method for assessing cortical excitability and inhibition in the motor cortex that has been applied to this disorder. If single-pulse TMS is given to the motor cortex while the subject maintains weak, voluntary tonic contractions of the stimulated muscle, a "silent period" is induced whereby the corresponding motor evoked potential is suppressed. In addition, if an initial, conditioning subthreshold TMS pulse is followed by a second suprathreshold test TMS pulse within 1–6 milliseconds, the amplitude of the motor evoked potential is reduced. Patients with writer's cramp have demonstrated reduced silent period and reduced paired-pulse inhibition, findings that suggest the existence of diminished intracortical inhibition in this disorder (Filipovic et al. 1997; Mavroudakis et al. 1995; Ridding et al. 1995). Such findings prompted Siebner et al. (1999) to examine whether 1-Hz rTMS to motor cortex could normalize impaired intracortical inhibition in this condition and improve handwriting. Active rTMS was found to increase corticocortical inhibition by the paired-pulse TMS method in the dystonic group but not in a control group without dystonia. In a second experiment, a total of 16 patients participated, including eight patients with simple writer's cramp and eight patients with dystonic writer's cramp. Quality of handwriting, handwriting pressure, and duration of post-TMS silent period during voluntary muscle contraction were assessed. Significant handwriting improvement lasting at least 3 hours after active rTMS was observed in eight patients. Two of these subjects reported improvement that persisted many days. Three of 10 patients reported some improvement after placebo/sham rTMS.

In some studies rTMS is being used to probe brain regions other than motor cortex in various illnesses. These illnesses include posttraumatic stress disorder (PTSD), obsessive-compulsive disorder (OCD), and schizophrenia.

Posttraumatic Stress Disorder

Grisaru et al. (1998) were the first to report results of a study in which patients with PTSD were treated with rTMS. In a study in which neither investigators nor subjects were masked, 10 patients received 0.3-Hz rTMS to both left and right motor cortex at maximum power of a stimulator (Magstim 200; Magstim, Whitland, Wales), 15 pulses to each. Symptoms of PTSD, such as avoidance, and overall clinical state according to the Clinical Global Impression (CGI) Scale transiently improved for 1–7 days after the rTMS session.

Two cases of PTSD studied with rTMS were described by McCann et al. (1998). The approach was based on the results of functional neuroimaging studies that suggested patients with PTSD have right-sided frontal activation (Rauch et al. 1996; Shin et al. 1997). Effects of open-label 1-Hz rTMS administered once daily for 17 days to one patient and for 30 days to a second patient were assessed. Both patients received rTMS to the right prefrontal cortex. The first patient had a previous trial of 20-Hz left prefrontal rTMS without symptomatic improvement. Both patients demonstrated improvements in symptoms that lasted approximately 1 month after the trial. Baseline neuroimaging of these two patients was conducted with fluorodeoxyglucose (FDG) PET, and scans were repeated after the trial. In both cases, decreased regional brain metabolism was detected. More prominent changes were found over the right hemisphere, the side of stimulation.

The results described by McCann et al. were consistent with those of a later rTMS study of effects of right versus left prefrontal 1-Hz rTMS in normal subjects. Behavioral effects were determined in response to angry faces during performance of an emotional face version of the Stroop task (D'Alfonso et al. 2000). Consistent with accounts of neural mechanisms of approach and withdrawal behaviors, right-sided stimulation inactivated avoidance reactions to angry faces, whereas left-sided stimulation had the opposite effect. Insofar as a symptom of PTSD is avoidance of perceived threat, these findings suggest that right prefrontal 1-Hz rTMS can reduce emotional reactivity in PTSD patients.

An open-label case series of 12 patients with comorbid PTSD and major depression was described by Rosenberg et al. (2002). Each subject received rTMS to left frontal cortex as an adjunct to antidepressant drugs at 90% of motor threshold, 1 Hz or 5 Hz, 6,000 stimuli over 10 days. Seventy-five percent of the patients were reported to have reduced depression symptoms after rTMS, with improvements in anxiety, hostility, and insomnia, but only minimal improvement in PTSD symptoms.

The results of the studies by McCann et al., D'Alfonso et al., and Rosenberg et al. were largely inconclusive. The protocol described by McCann et al. seemed the most promising insofar as it was guided by functional neuroimaging data. However, to the best of my knowledge, results of more recent studies of right prefrontal 1-Hz rTMS in PTSD patients have not been reported.

Obsessive-Compulsive Disorder

The first study examining rTMS effects in patients with OCD was described by Greenberg et al. (1997). The rationale for the study derived from results of previous studies demonstrating prefrontal hypermetabolism or hyperperfusion in patients with OCD (Hoehn-Saric and Benkelfat 1994). The investigators hoped that directly altering prefrontal activity by applying higher-frequency rTMS to prefrontal cortex would transiently interrupt OCD symptoms. Moreover, results of numerous studies have suggested antidepressant effects of such protocols. Findings that antidepressant medications reduce OCD symptoms suggest that the antidepressant effects of rTMS may reduce OCD symptoms in an analogous manner. Twelve right-handed patients with OCD diagnosed according to the DSM-III-R criteria (American Psychiatric Association 1987) participated in the study. Four received no medication, and eight continued to take stable doses of selective serotonin reuptake inhibitors. Six patients also met the DSM-III-R criteria for current or past major depression. Stimulation was applied to a left prefrontal site, a right prefrontal site, and a midline occipital site as an active control site. Stimulation was at 80% motor threshold for a single session each at 20 Hz, 2 seconds per minute for 20 minutes. Compulsive urges were reduced by right prefrontal stimulation up to 8 hours after stimulation. Left prefrontal stimulation and occipital stimulation did not produce these improvements. Of interest is that obsessive thoughts did not change significantly after any type of stimulation. Parallel though modest effects in mood also were detected. These effects of a single session of rTMS were admittedly transient, but they suggested that rTMS may provide a useful probe of neurocircuitry producing OCD symptoms.

Results of a second study of rTMS in the treatment of OCD patients were reported by Sachdev et al. (2001). Subjects were 12 right-handed persons meeting the DSM-IV (American Psychiatric Association 1994) criteria for OCD but not current criteria for major depression, although nine had comorbid histories of past depression. Patients were randomized to receive either left or right prefrontal rTMS. Stimulation parameters were 10 Hz, 30 trains of 5 seconds each, 25 seconds between trains, and 110% resting motor threshold. The trial lasted 10 weekdays. In this study, there were no significant differences in response to left versus right prefrontal stimulation. Statistically significant improvement according to the Yale-Brown Obsessive Compulsive Scale (YBOCS) was observed for both groups combined. Improvement was detected after the 2-week trial and at 1-month follow-up evaluation. Two (33%) of the six subjects in each group had clinically significant improvement (i.e., YBOCS score improved at least 40%). There was no control condition.

In a later study, Greenberg et al. (2000) examined cortical excitability in OCD patients. Sixteen patients with this disorder participated in the study. Nine of these patients received fluoxetine and seven patients were not treated with medication. Eleven healthy persons participated as a comparison group. In examination of motor thresholds in the two groups, the investigators found a significant reduction in the OCD group compared with the control subjects, an effect that was detected at a statistically significant level even when the analysis was restricted to the patient group not receiving medication. In addition, the paired-pulse paradigm showed reduced cortical inhibition in the OCD group. Once again, this effect was detected even when comparisons were limited to the patients not taking medication. These data suggested excessive excitability in OCD patients, at least in motor cortex.

Results of a sham-controlled rTMS trial with this patient group were reported by Alonso et al. (2001). Study participants were 18 right-handed persons meeting the DSM-IV criteria for OCD. Five subjects were not taking medication. No patient met the DSM-IV criteria for another Axis I disorder. Patients were randomly allocated to groups receiving right prefrontal rTMS or sham stimulation. The trial consisted of 18 sessions (three sessions per week for 6 weeks) at a frequency of 1 Hz of 20 minutes' duration and 110% motor threshold. Stimulation was performed with a circular coil positioned roughly over Brodmann area 9 and area 46 on the basis of extrapolation from magnetic resonance imaging (MRI) models of the head that were projected onto each patient's head with external landmarks. No significant changes in symptoms were detected for either group.

The negative results obtained by Alonso et al. (2001) are significant given that Greenberg et al. (2000) found increased cortical excitability, which suggested that 1-Hz "suppressive" rTMS should have had a symptom-reducing effect. These findings, considered together, suggest the use of low-frequency rTMS to reverse putative increases in cortical excitability is not always fruitful. A limitation of the findings of Greenberg et al. (2000) is that they refer to the motor cortex, which may not reflect properties of other cortical circuits directly involved in generation of OCD symptoms. In their study Sachdev et al. (2001) did not find robust clinical effects in most patients and did not find a laterality effect. Their data therefore seem to be partial disconfirmation of the results of the study by Greenberg et al. (1997). Of note, however, was that the latter study showed only transient effects of a single session of rTMS, which does not necessarily translate into sustained effects for an extended trial.

Schizophrenia

The first study of rTMS in patients with schizophrenia was described by Geller et al. (1997). The subjects were 10 patients with schizophrenia and 10 patients with depression. The study was conducted to determine whether mood changes could be induced. Very-low-frequency (once per 30 seconds) rTMS was administered to prefrontal cortex on the left and right sides with a total of 15 pulses administered to each side. Two of 10 schizophrenic patients appeared to have transient improvement. In a study in which neither subjects nor investigators were masked, Feinsod et al. (1998) found that 7 of 10 patients with schizophrenia experienced decreased anxiety and restlessness in response to low-frequency frontal rTMS. On the other hand, in a later, double-masked study of the effects of 1-Hz rTMS to right prefrontal cortex, Klein et al. (1999a) did not find any improvement after active stimulation relative to sham stimulation. This study was prompted by results of an earlier study demonstrating antidepressant effects with this stimulation protocol in patients with major depression (Klein et al. 1999b). The authors had sought to determine the specificity of these putative treatment effects by comparing results with those from another diagnostic group.

Rollnik et al. (2000), using a double-masked crossover design, examined the effects of higher-frequency rTMS delivered to left prefrontal cortex in 12 schizophrenic patients with negative symptoms. This approach was motivated by evidence suggesting that higher-frequency rTMS has an activating influence on cortical function (Post et al. 1997) and by results of other studies demonstrating hypofrontality in schizophrenia (Weinberger and Berman 1996). Left prefrontal rTMS was administered daily for 2 weeks. Each stimulation session consisted of 20 2-second pulse trains at 20 Hz and 80% motor threshold delivered to dorsolateral prefrontal cortex. The Brief Psychiatric Rating Scale score decreased after active rTMS ($P < 0.05$) compared with sham stimulation, whereas depressive and anxiety symptoms did not change significantly. Interestingly, symptom changes detected in this trial did not appear to reflect predominantly negative symptoms.

Yu et al. (2002) investigated effects of 10-Hz rTMS administered to left prefrontal cortex in five patients with schizophrenia. The main goal was to determine rTMS effects on P300 abnormalities and elevated prolactin levels induced by antipsychotic drugs. Partial normalization of each of these abnormalities was detected. Given that elevated prolactin level was likely due to dopamine blockade, partial normalization of prolactin suggests that a mechanism of action of prefrontal rTMS in the higher frequency range is enhanced dopaminergic function. These findings were consistent with those of a more recent TMS study with psychiatrically healthy subjects. In that study, after delivery of high-frequency rTMS to prefrontal cortex, raclopride C 11 PET showed evidence of increased dopamine release (Strafella et al. 2001).

Impairment of working memory in schizophrenia often has been linked to reduced activation in prefrontal areas (Barch et al. 2001; Goldman-Rakic 1999). In a study with psychiatrically healthy subjects, Yamanaka et al. (2002) found that brief exposures of 10-Hz rTMS over left prefrontal cortex produced temporary improvement in working memory. If similar effects can be obtained with higher-frequency rTMS to prefrontal cortex in patients with schizophrenia, not only overt symptoms but also core neuropsychological impairments may improve.

In a case series of six patients with chronic schizophrenia examined with rTMS, Cohen et al. (1999) began to consider these issues. All patients were taking a stable dose of antipsychotic medication and received 20-Hz rTMS, 10 sessions over 2 weeks, with 2-second pulse trains given once per minute for 20 minutes at 80% motor threshold. Neuropsychological testing and single-photon emission computed tomography (SPECT) were performed both at baseline and after the rTMS protocol. Negative symptoms, as measured by the Positive and Negative Syndrome Scale for Schizophrenia (PANSS), were observed to decline after rTMS to a degree that was statistically significant ($P < 0.05$). There was a trend toward neuropsychological improvement with significant improvement detected for the delayed visual memory task. No change in hypofrontality was detected on repeat SPECT scanning after rTMS.

The foregoing results, considered together, suggest that further rTMS studies of prefrontal function in schizophrenia have promise. Results of only one controlled study have been reported (Rollnik et al. 2000), so the previous results must be considered very preliminary.

Our research group has focused on auditory hallucinations. This symptom of schizophrenia occurs in 60% to 70% of cases and often produces severe distress, disability, and loss of behavioral control. In approximately 25% of patients, auditory hallucinations respond poorly or not at all to currently available antipsychotic medication (Shergill et al. 1998). One important feature of auditory hallucinations is that they generally are experienced as spoken speech with discernible loudness, timbre, and other "percept-like" features. These characteristics suggest direct involvement of speech perception neurocircuitry. Support for this view is derived from the observation that patients with hallucinated speech, compared with psychiatrically healthy subjects, are more likely to experience perceptual illusions of words or word phrases when listening to acoustic noise (Alpert 1985; Bentall and Slade 1985). These early findings suggest excessive sensitivity or reactivity of speech perception systems.

A computer neural network simulation of speech perception processes demonstrated that auditory hallucinations could arise from a loss of intrinsic connectivity within the working memory module of the network (Hoffman and McGlashan 1997). Simulation of this "lesion" was motivated by growing evidence suggesting the existence of reduced cortical connectivity in schizophrenia (see McGlashan and Hoffman 2000 for review) with special vulnerability involving intrinsic (i.e., within-module or intra-areal) connections (Lewis and Gonzalez-Burgos 2000). In this simulation, excessive pruning of connections in the working memory module caused subsets of neurons to coactivate autonomously—unbuffered by interactions with other neurons in the larger network. As a result, the system produced output in the absence of any input—thereby simulating hallucinated speech. With these computer simulation models, investigators predicted that patients with auditory hallucinations would also experience perceptual distortions when listening to spoken speech when acoustic clarity is reduced. This finding was confirmed in a later study in which schizophrenic patients with active auditory hallucinations, schizophrenic patients without hallucinations, and nonschizophrenic control subjects were compared (Hoffman et al. 1999a).

In some neuroimaging studies, investigators have detected activation in temporoparietal cortex during auditory hallucination periods (Lennox et al. 2000; Silbersweig et al. 1995). The temporoparietal cortex is adjacent to Wernicke's area and is active during speech perception (Benson et al. 2001). On the basis of results of studies demonstrating that 1-Hz rTMS produces sustained reduction in cortical activation (Chen et al. 1997; Wassermann et al. 1998), my colleagues and I predicted that 1-Hz rTMS might reduce auditory hallucinations. We targeted the left temporoparietal cortex on the basis of results of neuroimaging studies cited above (Lennox et al. 2000; Silbersweig et al. 1995). This brain area underlies verbal memory and semantic processing during speech perception (Fiez et al. 1996; Ojemann 1978)—specific functions our previous studies showed were malfunctioning in hallucinating patients (Hoffman and McGlashan 1997; Hoffman et al. 1999a). This area is readily accessible to scalp stimulation insofar as the depth of overlying skull and muscle is not prohibitive.

My colleagues and I initially reported results of a study in which the subjects were 12 right-handed schizophrenic patients with medication-resistant auditory hallucinations. Using a double-masked crossover design, we compared the effects of 1-Hz active rTMS with effects that occurred during sham stimulation (Hoffman et al. 1999a, 2000). All patients received either typical or atypical antipsychotic medication. Five patients received concomitant anticonvulsant medication (divalproex [$n=4$], carbamazepine [$n=1$]). All patients had experienced auditory hallucinations without remission for at least 6 months. Patients were excluded if they had a history of epilepsy or were currently treated with clozapine. Each patient was right-handed and had normal results of routine laboratory studies, electrocardiogram, and electroencephalogram.

Stimulation was administered at 80% of motor threshold with a Cadwell water-cooled figure-eight coil. Site of stimulation was exactly halfway between the left temporal (T3) and left parietal (P3) positions according to the International 10-20 electroencephalographic (EEG) system. The sham stimulation was administered to the same location with the coil tilted 45 degrees off the scalp in a double-wing position. Insofar as this study was the first in which rTMS was administered in this brain area, we were very cautious regarding patient safety and tolerability. The first day, the patient received 4 minutes of stimulation; this was increased in 4-minute increments to 16 minutes on the final, fourth day of that arm of the trial. An earlier study had revealed that severity of auditory hallucinations reflected a range of variables (e.g., frequency, loudness, content, number of voices, emotional distress, and level of distraction) that varied from one patient to the next. Consequently, auditory hallucinations were assessed with an individualized, composite scale that was anchored by the patient's self-report of symptoms of hallucinations at the start of the study. A score of 10 was assigned to this narrative description; a score of zero corresponded to no hallucinations and a score of 20 to hallucinations that were twice as severe as baseline. The PANSS was used for assessment of changes in other symptoms. Reassessment of hallucinations was performed the day after each rTMS session and reflected severity of hallucinations over the intervening time. Patients, clinical raters, and clinicians working with patients were masked regarding stimulation condition.

The first four patients in this study underwent EEG monitoring after each 4-minute block of rTMS. No EEG abnormalities were detected after rTMS in any of these patients, and this monitoring procedure was discontinued for later patients. Patients were monitored with two subtests of the Mini-Mental State Examination.

Besides some complaints of headache, patients tolerated rTMS without difficulty. No verbal memory or attentional impairments were detected, nor was there any evidence of speech perception or language difficulty.

Mean baseline hallucination scores for the active rTMS trial and the sham trial were not significantly different. A random-effects model was used to assess treatment effects of different stimulation times relative to baseline for each of the two stimulation conditions. Symptom improvement relative to baseline was not statistically significant for 4 or 8 minutes of active stimulation but was significant after 12 minutes of active stimulation ($P<0.03$) and after 16 minutes of active stimulation ($P<0.0001$) (Figure 2–1). Statistically significant clinical improvements were not detected for sham stimulation at any of the four durations. No effect of order of stimulation (active followed by sham versus sham followed by active) was detected. When endpoint data were compared, statistically significant improvements in auditory hallucinations were detected for active rTMS relative to sham stimulation ($P<0.01$) (Figure 2–2). Therapeutic effects were brief, generally lasting less than 1 week. Concomitant use of anticonvulsant medication was found to curtail the symptom-reducing effects of rTMS, an effect that was statistically significant ($P<0.02$) (see Figure 2–2). Insofar as anticonvulsant drugs limit transsynaptic propagation of cortical activation (Applegate et al. 1997), these data suggest that putative therapeutic effects of rTMS require propagation of activation between neurons. Other positive symptoms of schizophrenia were relatively unchanged by rTMS, a finding that suggests protocol effects were relatively selective.

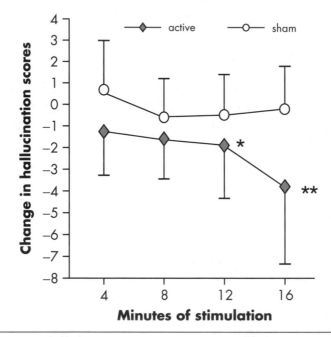

Figure 2–1. Hallucination severity ratings reflecting symptoms assessed the day after repetitive transcranial magnetic stimulation at the duration shown.

Y axis reflects changes in severity relative to baseline for active and sham stimulation trials. Data were analyzed by using a random effects model with Dunnett's criterion to adjust for multiple comparisons. Error bars represent standard deviations.

*t=2.3, df=44, P<0.03.

** t=4.7, df=44, P<0.0001.

Source. From Hoffman RE, Boutros NN, Hu S, et al.: "Transcranial Magnetic Stimulation and Auditory Hallucinations in Schizophrenia." *The Lancet* 355:1073–1075, 2000 (p. 1074). Reprinted with permission from Elsevier Science.

We consequently sought to determine whether a more extended trial of rTMS administered to left temporoparietal cortex could produce more clinically significant reductions in auditory hallucinations. This study has again focused on patients whose auditory hallucinations have proved resistant to currently available antipsychotic medication. We have reported results for the first 24 patients with medication-resistant hallucinations enrolled in this trial (Hoffman et al. 2003). All subjects were right-handed and demonstrated medication resistance on the basis of

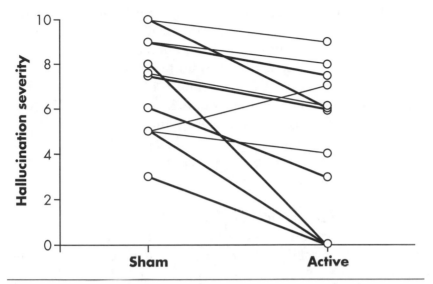

Figure 2–2. Endpoint auditory hallucination severity for sham versus active rTMS in patients receiving concomitant anticonvulsant medication (*thin rule*) and patients not receiving anticonvulsant medication (*heavy rule*).

Source. From Hoffman RE, Boutros NN, Hu S, et al.: "Transcranial Magnetic Stimulation and Auditory Hallucinations in Schizophrenia." *The Lancet* 355:1073–1075, 2000 (p. 1074). Reprinted with permission from Elsevier Science.

objective criteria (unsuccessful trials of two antipsychotic drugs of at least 6 weeks at therapeutic dosages, at least one drug being an atypical agent). In a study with a double-masked, parallel design, patients were randomized to receive either active ($n=12$) or sham ($n=12$) treatment. There were no statistically significant differences between groups in terms of age, sex, number of previous hospitalizations, or duration of current hallucination episode. Length of time of unremitting hallucinations tended to be very extended, a mean of roughly 10 years in each group. No change in dose of antipsychotic or thymoleptic medication was made for 4 weeks before trial entry and during the trial itself. Study participants, clinical raters, and all personnel responsible for the clinical care of the participants remained masked to allocated condition. A Magstim Super system with a figure-eight 70-mm coil was used. As in our first study, 1-Hz stimulation was administered halfway between T3 and P3, according to the International 10-20 EEG system, but with a higher field strength (90% motor threshold versus 80% in our first study). Patients in this trial received 8 minutes of stimulation on day 1, 12 minutes of stimulation on day 2, and 16 minutes of stimulation for the next 7 days (excluding weekends) for a total of 132 minutes of stimulation (compared with 40 minutes for our first trial). Neuropsychological assessments were administered at baseline, during the trial, and at the end of each arm of the trial. Patients were assessed with the Auditory Hallucinations Rating Scale developed by our group, the PANSS, and the CGI-Improvement scale.

Patients in general tolerated the trial without difficulty. Two patients dropped out of the study because of clinical deterioration, both during the sham arm of the trial. One patient was removed from the study during the active arm after development of angina-like chest pain and electrocardiographic changes. Insofar as the patient had significant risk factors (smoking and diabetes mellitus), this complication appeared unrelated to rTMS. There was no statistical evidence that rTMS produced cognitive decline. There was a significant time effect ($P<0.0001$) and a significant time by treatment interaction ($P<0.003$) for overall hallucination severity in the double-masked phase of the trial. These findings reflected greater improvement during the active trial compared with the sham trial. Aspects of hallucinatory experience that improved most robustly were frequency and attentional salience of hallucinations. The latter variable reflected the degree that hallucinations co-opted attention in terms of their disruptive effects on thought and behavior. Although no other specific groups of symptoms consistently improved, overall well-being of the patients as reflected by CGI showed more improvement for patients in the active arm than for those in the sham arm of the study in endpoint scores (mean±SD) for the active double-masked group ($P=0.006$). Follow-up assessment revealed that duration of improvement ranged between 1 week and more than 1 year, approximately one-half of the patients retaining improvements 4 months after the trial.

Our findings highlight the likely involvement of the left temporoparietal area in generation of auditory hallucinations. Insofar as our site of stimulation—left temporoparietal cortex—is strongly implicated in receptive language processing (Benson et al. 2001), these findings are evidence that auditory hallucinations arise, at least in part, from these physiological systems. Given that improvements after active rTMS often appeared to be clinically significant (9 of 12 patients had at least 50% improvement in hallucinations compared with 2 of 12 patients in the sham treatment group), further study of 1-Hz rTMS as treatment of this indication appears warranted.

One attempt to replicate our findings was reported (d'Alfonso et al. 2002). Eight patients with persistent auditory hallucinations were given an open-label trial of 1-Hz rTMS. Stimulation was at 80% motor threshold at somewhat longer duration of 20 minutes of stimulation per day for 10 days. Statistically significant improvements in auditory hallucinations were detected, although improvements were relatively modest. Possible explanations for reduced response include the fact that one of the 8 patients was left-handed. There is therefore an approximately 50% chance that this patient could have been right-hemisphere dominant, which could reduce effects of rTMS administered to the left hemisphere. Moreover, another patient needed a reduction in stimulation from 80% to 50% because of pain at the site of stimulation, which also may have significantly reduced rTMS effects. Third, stimulation in this study was not administered to left temporoparietal cortex but to a left temporal region 2 cm above T3 according to the International 10/20 system. Given that the T3 site tends to overlap the superior and middle temporal gyrus (Homan et al. 1987), it is possible that 2-cm displacement in a superior direction could move the stimulation coil off the temporal lobe to a functionally unrelated region in some cases. We also found that a subgroup of hallucinating patients has no improvement after active rTMS to our "standard" left temporoparietal site. These are patients whose auditory hallucinations are constant and unremitting during wakefulness. This subgroup of hallucinators report special phenomenological features, including tinnitus, marked worsening of hallucinations in response to external sounds, and multiple overlapping "voices" heard as a continuous "mumble," often without discernible content. These phenomenological characteristics suggest greater involvement of primary auditory cortex rather than Wernicke's area during auditory hallucinations. Inclusion of such patients in studies will tend to reduce observed rTMS effects.

Where the rTMS coil is positioned for these trials is a critical variable. The optimum location may not be the same from one patient to the next given that the anatomical distribution of language functions normally can vary considerably across individuals (Ojemann 1991). We consequently have initiated an rTMS trial in which location of magnetic stimulation is directed by topographic location of functional MRI (fMRI) data used to probe neurocircuitry involvement underlying auditory hallucinations. In three cases, activation maps of hallucination periods were generated by having patients depress a button during scanning for the duration of individual episodes of hallucinations. T-maps of hallucination periods compared with nonhallucination periods were generated. An alternative method for mapping functionally engaged neurocircuitry was developed for three additional patients whose hallucinations were constant during wakefulness. In these cases, there were no nonhallucination periods during fMRI that could be used as a comparison condition to delineate hallucination-specific activation. For these cases correlation maps relative to Wernicke's area were generated for blood oxygenation level–dependent (BOLD) signal fluctuations during scanning periods when there was external silence. Results have indicated that BOLD correlation maps delineate functional connectivity between cortical regions (Cordes et al. 2000; Hampson et al. 2002; Lowe et al. 2000). Our assumption is that auditory hallucinations involve activity in Wernicke's region—but also in other brain regions, such as Broca's region, that are functionally connected to Wernicke's region. A frameless stereotactic system (BrainLAB, Munich, Germany) was used to identify scalp locations corresponding to underlying regions of interest. rTMS was administered to three regions identified with fMRI maps plus a sham stimulation region based on these data. Each site received 3 days of 1-Hz stimulation of 16 minutes' duration each at 90% motor threshold. Four of six patients had a clinical response in this fMRI-guided protocol. Comparison with results from our rTMS trial in which standard temporoparietal placement was used suggested that fMRI-based placement of rTMS enhances efficacy in reducing auditory hallucinations (R. Hoffman, R. Buchanan, A. Anderson, M. Hampson, K. Wu, N. Boutros, J. Gore, D. Spencer, J. Krystal, unpublished data, November 2002). A larger sample of patients is needed for rigorous testing of this hypothesis.

Our findings with low-frequency rTMS targeting speech processing areas are further evidence that speech perception neurocircuitry participates in generation of auditory hallucinations, one of the most vexing and resistant symptoms associated with schizophrenia. The possible clinical utility of these results awaits further study. Foremost is the issue of duration of effects. For patients in the Hoffman et al. (2003) trial, 9/12 of those randomly assigned to the sham condition subsequently received an open-label trial of active rTMS to a single, left temporoparietal site. Pooling those receiving both types of active rTMS, 11/21 patients retained significant improvement after 14 weeks, and 5/21 patients retained improvement at 1 year. We have now begun to re-enroll patients with reoccurrence of symptoms in a more extended, open-label trial (consisting of a total of 192 minutes of stimulation over 12 days versus 132 minutes over 9 days in our current trial) to that same site. The first five patients have shown brisk improvement in auditory hallucinations and other symptoms when patients were re-exposed to rTMS—but roughly the same duration of improvement as in our standard protocol. Thus it appears that more extended rTMS may not prolong duration of improvement. If so, the next step is to undertake a maintenance trial for these patients in which rTMS is given 1 or 2 times per week in order to sustain improvement. These research efforts will have to include high-level monitoring with neuropsychological testing to ensure that extended exposure to 1-Hz rTMS over many weeks does not induce deficits. Our paramount concern in conducting these trials is safety and tolerability. This concern is underscored by the fact that patients with schizophrenia have preexisting cognitive impairments, which can cause them to be more vulnerable to additional cognitive impairment.

Conclusion

A number of issues must be considered in evaluating the studies described in this chapter. First, many of these studies are conducted without a sham or placebo control condition. It is common for intervention development to be initiated with uncontrolled case series, and the results can be a useful guide in selecting promising research directions. However, without adequate controls and sizable samples, it is impossible to determine whether a putative treatment has clinical benefit. The idea of placing a magnet on someone's head to alter symptoms is a potent concept for many persons, and increased hopefulness and other suggestion effects—which are not to be underestimated—are likely to come into play. Therefore all studies that are open label must be considered in that light. Even reports such as that of McCann et al. (1998)—in which symptom improvements were accompanied by neuroimaging changes in the direction of normalization—must be considered in terms of possible placebo effects, which can improve mood, reduce anxiety, and diminish hopelessness. These changes in emotional state and attitude are likely to have correlates in terms of neurobiological function. In some sense, the most useful results of open-label case series are negative results—if results of a study do not suggest possible clinical efficacy under these conditions, it is less likely that a similar protocol will produce evidence of clinical efficacy when compared with control stimulation. Unfortunately, negative results are often not reported in the literature.

The challenge of developing an effective placebo-like control condition for rTMS is not simple. There is some suggestion that the usual method of delivering sham stimulation—tipping the stimulation coil 45 degrees off the scalp—can retain some biological effects if both wings of the figure-eight coil remain in contact with the scalp (Loo et al. 2000). Another factor to consider is that the somatic sensations (such as scalp muscle contractions or a "knocking" sensation) of sham stimulation may be less than that produced by active stimulation. In crossover studies patients have a chance to mentally compare the two conditions and may be able to guess that the condition with the stronger sensation is the active condition. This was a potential limitation of our first rTMS study of auditory hallucinations, although we did use the double-wing tilt position for sham stimulation. After our second trial, we debriefed each patient regarding their best guess regarding type of simulation and the basis for the guess. The guesses were often correct, but inevitably they were reported to be based on clinical response rather than degree of somatic sensation. I believe that in the long run, sham control methods commonly used for rTMS studies are at least as good, in terms of somatic cueing, as those in most central nervous system pharmacological studies in which the placebo agent is inert and lacks side effects that commonly occur with the active agent.

An alternative is to use an active stimulation comparison site. Motor cortex as a comparison region might be considered for such stimulation. However, this region has a lower seizure threshold. Therefore rTMS to this region is likely to have a somewhat higher risk of seizure induction. For that reason our group has avoided this strategy. It is less clear whether other sites, at least for patients with schizophrenia, are truly uninvolved in the mechanisms of the disorder, especially because rTMS has effects propagated from the site of stimulation to other functionally active brain regions. Finally, control stimulation to another region may have unknown risk in terms of cognitive impairment, especially in populations already known to have cognitive deficits. Another obvious limitation of sham or active control stimulation is that the person administering the rTMS is not masked. Hence there must be rigorous efforts to restrict interaction between the person administering rTMS and other personnel involved with the study, as well as the patient, during the trial. Sham coils that look identical to active coils are under development to help solve the problem of investigator masking.

The assumption that higher-frequency rTMS is activating and lower-frequency rTMS is deactivating is likely to be only a rough approximation of actual rTMS effects. Much remains to be learned about rTMS effects in the brain (Post and Keck 2001). A number of studies with rodents have been conducted with promising results. For instance, higher-frequency rTMS has demonstrated complex alterations of neurocircuitry function in the hippocampus that appear similar to those induced by antidepressant drugs (Levkovitz et al. 2001).

There is growing interest in considering rTMS from the vantage point of neuroplasticity (Post et al. 1997). For example, 20-Hz rTMS in rodents has been shown to induce release of brain-derived neurotrophic factor (Post and Keck 2001). This factor plays an important role in regulating and maintaining connectivity in neural networks. Moreover, low-frequency rTMS may have neuroplastic effects analogous to the long-term depotentiation elicited experimentally by direct, selective electrical stimulation of the brain in animal studies (Hoffman and Cavus 2002). This neuroplastic effect selectively reverses synaptic modifications that have been strengthened by experimentally induced LTP while leaving unchanged other components of synaptic efficacy.

It is possible that LTP provides a pathological model. If so, long-term depotentiation may have special utility in selective attenuation of pathologically reinforced network interactions while leaving normal brain function intact. These comments notwithstanding, there is much that we do not understand about effects of rTMS. For example, in studies with rodents, investigators are unable to recreate the selective effects of rTMS when stimulation is administered to specific brain regions. Studies with primates, in which rTMS can be administered more selectively, are under way.

My expectation is that the success of rTMS treatment studies of the sort described in this chapter will require further advances in our understanding of the functional anatomy and pathophysiology of psychiatric disorders and application of these insights in designing rTMS intervention trials. In numerous functional neuroimaging studies of schizophrenia, depression, PTSD, and OCD, investigators have documented under- and over-activation in a range of cortical and subcortical regions. However, our understanding of illness mechanisms remains very limited unless we address why these findings occur and how they are translated into the characteristic signs and symptoms of the disorder in question. Along these lines, our original view that hallucinated speech arises simply from activation of posterior speech-processing brain areas has been replaced by a more complex model. Our more recent hypothesis is that auditory hallucinations arise from excessive coupling between speech-generation areas of the brain (such as Broca's area) and posterior speech-perception brain areas (such Wernicke's region). Broca's area consequently may "dump" language outputs into the Wernicke's region, producing spontaneous, hallucinated speech percepts. Consequently rTMS intervention in our fMRI-guided protocol is now directed at an anatomically distributed network rather than a single brain area.

Another example of how functional neuroimaging can be used to guide rTMS trials is an rTMS trial undertaken in our laboratory (led by Dr. Adrian Preda in collaboration Drs. Mark George and Ziad Nahas, Medical University of South Carolina) that probes the pathophysiology of borderline personality disorder. This approach is based on other work at Yale University demonstrating that during fMRI examinations, patients with this disorder exhibit excessive neurobiological reactivity in response to faces expressing negative emotion. Excessive reactivity was observed in the left amygdala and a prefrontal region, the location of which varied somewhat from patient to patient (Donegan et al. 2002). Our intervention strategy was to target these patient-specific prefrontal areas to access an anatomically distributed "emotion" network with suppressive 1-Hz rTMS. Thus far, the trial has included only seven patients, but preliminary data suggest that the active trial leads to reduced dysphoria in comparison with sham stimulation.

Results of one study suggest an alternative, neurobiologically informed rTMS strategy for PTSD patients (Milad and Quirk 2002). In a study with rats, a tone was paired to a fear response elicited by an electrical shock—the tone, when delivered alone, produced a fear response consisting of behavioral "freezing." If the tone was subsequently administered repeatedly to the rat, this fear response diminished, a process known as *extinction*. The degree of activation of neurons in the medial prefrontal cortex correlated positively with the animal's likelihood of extinguishing this fear response to a previously conditioned stimulus. Lesions in this brain area eliminated extinction of response to the tones, a finding that suggested a specific extinction memory is stored, at least in part, in the medial prefrontal cortex. The findings also showed that the conditioned stimulus, when paired with brief electrical stimulation of this brain region, produced extinction of the fear response. The authors suggested that consolidation of extinction learning potentiates neuronal activity, which inhibits fear during subsequent encounters with fear stimuli. This postulate is consistent with results of studies with PTSD patients in which correlations were found between increased autonomic arousal and depressed medial prefrontal activation when the subjects responded to cues reminding them of their traumatic memories (Bremner 2002; Shin et al. 2001). The authors suggested it may be possible to use higher-frequency rTMS directed at medial prefrontal cortex—analogous to direct electrical stimulation in rodent studies—to extinguish response to cues that ordinarily trigger a fear response in these patients. In other words, high-frequency rTMS to medial prefrontal cortex may mobilize extinction memories that selectively block retrieval of traumatic memories elicited by associated cues.

Despite the caveats, I remain optimistic that rTMS can be useful for testing illness models in neuropsychiatry. Through these efforts, we should be able to suggest fruitful strategies for developing alternative somatic treatments. I have found such research efforts to yield a kind of investigative bootstrapping, whereby rTMS efforts guide and inform new models of psychopathology, which lead to refinements in rTMS protocols. It is also possible that rTMS interventions will yield useful synergies with specific pharmacological and psychological treatments. For the very severe disorders discussed in this chapter, we need to be guided by other branches of medicine, such as oncology. For the near future, the most important research goal in terms of intervention development may be not discovery of a single definitive treatment but delineation of treatment combinations that maximize clinical outcome.

References

Alonso P, Pujol J, Cardoner N, et al: Right prefrontal repetitive transcranial magnetic stimulation in obsessive-compulsive disorder: a double-blind, placebo-controlled study. Am J Psychiatry 158:1143–1145, 2001

Alpert M: The signs and symptoms of schizophrenia. Compr Psychiatry 26:103–112, 1985

American Psychiatric Association: Diagnostic and Statistical Manual of Mental Disorders, 3rd Edition, Revised. Washington, DC, American Psychiatric Association, 1987

American Psychiatric Association: Diagnostic and Statistical Manual of Mental Disorders, 4th Edition. Washington, DC, American Psychiatric Association, 1994

Applegate CD, Samoriski GM, Ozduman K: Effects of valproate, phenytoin, and MK-801 in a novel model of epileptogenesis. Epilepsia 38:631–636, 1997

Barch DM, Carter CS, Braver TS, et al: Selective deficits in prefrontal cortex function in medication-naive patients with schizophrenia. Arch Gen Psychiatry 58:280–288, 2001

Benson RR, Whalen DH, Richardson M, et al: Parametrically dissociating speech and nonspeech perception in the brain using fMRI. Brain Lang 78:364–396, 2001

Bentall RP, Slade PD: Reality testing and auditory hallucinations. Br J Clin Psychol 24:159–169, 1985

Boroojerdi B, Prager A, Muelibacher W, et al: Reduction of human visual cortex excitability using 1-Hz transcranial magnetic stimulation. Neurology 11:1529–1531, 2000

Bremner JD: Neuroimaging studies in post-traumatic stress disorder. Curr Psychiatry Rep 4:254–263, 2002

Chen R, Classen J, Gerloff C, et al: Depression of motor cortex excitability by low-frequency transcranial magnetic stimulation. Neurology 48:1398–1403, 1997

Cohen E, Bernardo M, Masana J, et al: Repetitive transcranial magnetic stimulation in the treatment of chronic negative schizophrenia: a pilot study (letter). J Neurol Neurosurg Psychiatry 67:129–130, 1999

Cordes D, Haughton VM, Arfanakis K, et al: Mapping functionally related regions of brain with functional connectivity MR imaging. Am J Neuroradiol 21:1636–1644, 2000

D'Alfonso AA, van Honk J, Hermans E, et al: Laterality effects in selective attention to threat after repetitive transcranial stimulation at the prefrontal cortex in female subjects. Neurosci Lett 280:195–198, 2000

D'Alfonso AA, Aleman A, Kessels RP, et al: Transcranial magnetic stimulation of left auditory cortex in patients with schizophrenia: effects on hallucinations and neurocognition. J Neuropsychiatry Clin Neurosci 14:77–79, 2002

Donegan NH, Sanislow CA, Fulbright RK, et al: An fMRI study of the neural substrates of emotional dysregulation in borderline personality disorder (BPD). Program No. 498.2. 2002 Abstract Viewer/Itinerary Planner. Washington, DC, Society for Neuroscience, 2002. Available at: http://sfn.scholarone.com/itin2002/main.html?new_page_id=126& abstract_id=16941&p_num=498.2

Feinsod M, Kreinin B, Chistyakov A, et al: Preliminary evidence for a beneficial effect of low-frequency, repetitive transcranial magnetic stimulation in patients with major depression and schizophrenia. Depress Anxiety 7:65–68, 1998

Fiez JA, Raichle ME, Balota DA, et al: PET activation of posterior temporal regions during auditory word presentation and verb generation. Cereb Cortex 6:1–10, 1996

Filipovic SR, Ljubisavljevic M, Svetal M, et al: Impairment of cortical inhibition in writer's cramp as revealed by changes in electromyographic silent period after transcranial magnetic stimulation. Neurosci Lett 222:167–170, 1997

Geller V, Grisaru N, Abarbanel JM, et al: Slow magnetic stimulation of prefrontal cortex in depression and schizophrenia. Prog Neuropsychopharmacol Biol Psychiatry 21:105–110, 1997

Goldman-Rakic PS: The physiological approach: functional architecture of working memory and disordered cognition in schizophrenia. Biol Psychiatry 46:650–661, 1999

Greenberg BD, George MS, Martin JD, et al: Effect of prefrontal repetitive transcranial magnetic stimulation in obsessive-compulsive disorder: a preliminary study. Am J Psychiatry 154:867–869, 1997

Greenberg BD, Ziemann U, Cora-Locatelli G, et al: Altered cortical excitability in obsessive-compulsive disorder. Neurology 54:142–147, 2000

Grisaru N, Amir M, Cohen H, Kaplan Z: Effect of transcranial magnetic stimulation in posttraumatic stress disorder: a preliminary study. Biol Psychiatry 44:52–55, 1998

Hampson M, Peterson B, Skudlarski P, et al: Detection of functional connectivity using temporal correlations in MR images. Hum Brain Mapp 15:247–262, 2002

Hoehn-Saric R, Benkelfat C: Structural and functional brain imaging in OCD, in Current Concepts in OCD. Edited by Hollander E, Zohar J, Marazzati D. New York, Wiley, 1994, pp 183–211

Hoffman RE, Cavus I: Slow transcranial magnetic stimulation, long-term depotentiation, and brain hyperexcitability disorders. Am J Psychiatry 159:1093–1102, 2002

Hoffman RE, McGlashan TH: Synaptic elimination, neurodevelopment, and the mechanism of hallucinated "voices" in schizophrenia. Am J Psychiatry 154:1683–1688, 1997

Hoffman RE, Boutros NN, Berman RM, et al: Transcranial magnetic stimulation of left temporoparietal cortex in three patients reporting hallucinated "voices." Biol Psychiatry 46:130–132, 1999a

Hoffman RE, Rapaport J, Mazure CM, et al: Schizophrenic patients reporting hallucinated "voices" demonstrate selective speech perception alterations. Am J Psychiatry 156:393–399, 1999b

Hoffman RE, Boutros NN, Hu S, et al: Transcranial magnetic stimulation and auditory hallucinations in schizophrenia. Lancet 355:1073–1075, 2000

Hoffman RE, Hawkins KA, Gueorguieva R, et al: Transcranial magnetic stimulation of left temporoparietal cortex and medication-resistant auditory hallucinations. Arch Gen Psychiatry 60:49–56, 2003

Homan RW, Herman J, Purdy P: Cerebral location of International 10–20 system electrode replacement. Electroencephalogr Clin Neurophysiol 66:376–382, 1987

Klein E, Kolsky Y, Puyerovsky M, et al: Right prefrontal slow repetitive transcranial magnetic stimulation in schizophrenia: a double-blind sham-controlled pilot study. Biol Psychiatry 46:1451–1454, 1999a

Klein E, Kreinin I, Chistyakov A, et al: Therapeutic efficacy of right prefrontal slow repetitive transcranial magnetic stimulation in major depression: a double-blind controlled study. Arch Gen Psychiatry 56:315–320, 1999b

Lennox BR, Park SB, Medley I, et al: The functional anatomy of auditory hallucinations in schizophrenia. Psychiatry Res 100:13–20, 2000

Levkovitz Y, Grisaru N, Segal M: Transcranial magnetic stimulation and antidepressive drugs share similar cellular effects in rat hippocampus. Neuropsychopharmacology 24:608–616, 2001

Lewis DA, Gonzalez-Burgos G: Intrinsic excitatory connections in the prefrontal cortex and the pathophysiology of schizophrenia. Brain Res Bull 52:309–317, 2000

Loo CK, Taylor JL, Gandevia SC, et al: Transcranial magnetic stimulation (TMS) in controlled treatment studies: are some "sham" forms active? Biol Psychiatry 47:325–331, 2000

Lowe MJ, Dzemidzic M, Lurito JT, et al: Correlations in low-frequency BOLD fluctuations reflect cortico-cortical connections. Neuroimage 12:582–587, 2000

Mavroudakis N, Caroyer JM, Brunko E, et al: Abnormal motor evoked responses to transcranial magnetic stimulation in focal dystonia. Neurology 45:1671–1677, 1995

McCann UD, Kimbrell TA, Morgan CM, et al: Repetitive transcranial magnetic stimulation for posttraumatic stress disorder (letter). Arch Gen Psychiatry 55:277–279, 1998

McGlashan TH, Hoffman RE: Schizophrenia as a disorder of developmentally reduced synaptic connectivity. Arch Gen Psychiatry 57:637–648, 2000

Milad MR, Quirk GJ: Neurons in medial prefrontal cortex signal memory for fear extinction. Nature 420:70–74, 2002

Ojemann GA: Organization of short-term verbal memory of human cortex: evidence from electrical stimulation. Brain Lang 5:331–340, 1978

Ojemann GA: Cortical organization of language. J Neurosci 11:2281–2287, 1991

Pascual-Leone A, Valls-Sole J, Wassermann EM, et al: Responses to rapid-rate transcranial magnetic stimulation of the human motor cortex. Brain 117:847–858, 1994

Post A, Keck ME: Transcranial magnetic stimulation as a therapeutic tool in psychiatry: what do we know about neurobiological mechanisms? J Psychiatr Res 35:193–215, 2001

Post RM, Kimbrell, Frye M, et al: Implications of kindling and quenching for the possible frequency dependence of rTMS. CNS Spectr 2:54–60, 1997

Rauch SL, van der Kolk BA, Fisler RE, et al: A symptom provocation study of post-traumatic stress disorder using positron emission tomography and script-driven imagery. Arch Gen Psychiatry 53:380–387, 1996

Ridding MC, Sheean G, Rothwell JC, et al: Changes in the balance between motor cortical excitation and inhibition in focal, task specific dystonia. J Neurol Neurosurg Psychiatry 59:493–498, 1995

Rollnik JD, Huber TJ, Mogk H, et al: High-frequency repetitive transcranial magnetic stimulation (rTMS) of the dorsolateral prefrontal cortex in schizophrenic patients. Neuroreport 11:4013–4015, 2000

Rosenberg PB, Mehndiratta RB, Mehndiratta YP, et al: Repetitive transcranial magnetic stimulation treatment of comorbid posttraumatic stress disorder and major depression. J Neuropsychiatry Clin Neurosci 14:270–276, 2002

Rossi S, Pasqualetti P, Rossini PM, et al: Effects of repetitive transcranial magnetic stimulation on movement-related cortical activity in humans. Cereb Cortex 10:802–808, 2000

Sachdev PS, McBride R, Mitchell PB, et al: Right versus left prefrontal transcranial magnetic stimulation for obsessive-compulsive disorder: a preliminary investigation. J Clin Psychiatry 62:981–984, 2001

Shergill SS, Murray RM, McGuire PK: Auditory hallucinations: a review of psychological treatments. Schizophr Res 32:137–150, 1998

Shin LM, Kosslyn SM, McNally RJ, et al: Visual imagery and perception in posttraumatic stress disorder. Arch Gen Psychiatry 54:233–243, 1997

Shin LM, Whalen PJ, Pitman RK, et al: An fMRI study of anterior cingulate function in posttraumatic stress disorder. Biol Psychiatry 50:932–942, 2001

Siebner HR, Tormos JM, Ceballos-Baumann AO, et al: Low-frequency repetitive transcranial magnetic stimulation of the motor cortex in writer's cramp. Neurology 52:529–537, 1999

Silbersweig DA, Stern E, Frith C, et al: A functional neuroanatomy of hallucinations in schizophrenia. Nature 378:176–179, 1995

Speer AM, Kimbrell TA, Wassermann EM, et al: Opposite effects of high and low frequency rTMS on regional brain activity in depressed patients. Biol Psychiatry 48:1133–1141, 2000

Strafella AP, Paus T, Barrett J, et al: Repetitive transcranial magnetic stimulation of the human prefrontal cortex induces dopamine release in the caudate nucleus. J Neurosci 21:RC157, 2001

Wassermann EM, Wedegaertner FR, Ziemann UI, et al: Crossed reduction of human motor cortex excitability by 1-Hz transcranial magnetic stimulation. Neurosci Lett 250:141–144, 1998

Wedegaertner FR, Garvey MA, Cohen LG, et al: Low frequency repetitive transcranial magnetic stimulation can reduce action myoclonus (abstract). Neurology 48:A119, 1997

Weinberger DR, Berman KF: Prefrontal function in schizophrenia: confounds and controversies. Philos Trans R Soc Lond B Biol Sci 351:1495–1503, 1996

Yamanaka K, Li X, Nahas ZH, et al: Can prefrontal transcranial magnetic stimulation transiently improve working memory? In New Research Program and Abstracts, American Psychiatric Association 155th Annual Meeting, Philadelphia, PA, May 18–23, 2002, NR 131 (CD-ROM). Washington, DC, American Psychiatric Association, 2002

Yu H-C, Liao K-K, Chang T-J, et al: Transcranial magnetic stimulation in schizophrenia (letter). Am J Psychiatry 159:494–495, 2002

Chapter 3

Deep Brain Stimulation in Psychiatry

Benjamin D. Greenberg, M.D., Ph.D.

Techniques for direct or indirect alteration of the electrical activity of the brain are being developed as therapies in psychiatry. These brain stimulation techniques have different initial mechanisms of action. Electroconvulsive therapy delivers current to the brain across the large electrical resistance of the scalp and skull. Repetitive transcranial magnetic stimulation (rTMS) and magnetic seizure therapy induce electrical currents in brain tissue through an electromagnetic coil on the scalp. In vagus nerve stimulation, the vagus nerve in the neck is stimulated to affect its afferent projection targets and related brain circuits.

In deep brain stimulation (DBS), brain regions are directly stimulated with electrodes implanted within the brain. Over the past 15 years, DBS has been developed to the point that it has been approved by the U.S. Food and Drug Administration as a treatment for intractable movement disorders, currently tremor (Deuschl and Bain 2002; Schuurman et al. 2000; Tasker 1998) and Parkinson's disease (Pollak et al. 2002). The availability and technical refinement of this technique have opened a new avenue for research and possibly for treatment of severe and treatment-refractory neuropsychiatric disorders. The success of this therapy in treatment of Parkinson's disease and essential tremor has

This work is supported by an Independent Investigator Award from the National Alliance for Research on Schizophrenia and Depression to Dr. Greenberg and by research funding from Medtronic, Inc. Adapted with permission from "Mechanisms and State of the Art of Deep Brain Stimulation in Neuropsychiatry" *CNS Spectrums* 8(7):522–526, 2003.

spurred renewed interest in the use of such procedures for treatment of other refractory neurologic conditions. Neurologic illnesses for which DBS is under investigation include epilepsy (Hodaie et al. 2002; Loddenkemper et al. 2001), pain (Kumar et al. 1997), dystonia (Vercueil et al. 2002; Volkmann and Benecke 2002), and brain injury and persistent vegetative state (Schiff et al. 2002; Yamamoto et al. 2002). These and other possible indications anticipated from current research were reviewed by Mogilner et al. (2002).

In current practice, patients with tremor and Parkinson's disease who are potential candidates for this treatment have severe illness that has proved refractory to the best conventional medication therapies. For such patients, neurosurgical intervention is a therapeutic option. Modern stereotactic neurosurgery takes two forms: an ablative procedure or a neuromodulation approach with DBS. Use of lesion procedures in severe movement disorders has a long history (as it does in neuropsychiatry). The development of DBS, particularly the targets selected, followed that of the lesion procedures. At the same time, increasing understanding of the anatomical networks underlying pathophysiology of movement disorders was available to inform research on DBS as an investigational treatment. Coming full circle, the therapeutic effectiveness of DBS in movement disorders has opened a new window on these brain circuits and their potential roles in pathogenesis.

Therapeutic effectiveness of DBS in movement disorders has been well established. Benefit to quality of life as related to health also has been found (Just and Ostergaard 2002). Numerous reports have demonstrated the safety and efficacy of DBS surgery for intractable movement disorders. Studies of the outcome of DBS of the subthalamic nucleus and internal segment of the globus pallidus for Parkinson's disease have shown overall improvements of 41%–67% in standardized ratings of motor symptoms (Limousin et al. 1998; Vingerhoets et al. 2002; Voges et al. 2002; Volkmann et al. 2001). The results of thalamic stimulation for intractable tremor show that up to 85% of patients had significant improvements in their Parkinson's symptoms or essential tremor (Koller et al. 1997; Kumar et al. 1999; Limousin et al. 1998).

Surgical Implantation

Modern stereotactic techniques combine multiple imaging modalities, physiological mapping, and a high-speed surgical navigation computer for targeting any intracranial structure with millimeter precision (Rezai et al. 1997). Subcortical nuclei such as the globus pallidus internal segment, subthalamic nucleus, and thalamic nuclei are routinely localized during functional surgical procedures for Parkinson's disease, essential tremor, and dystonia. Anatomical localization is achieved with stereotactic imaging via magnetic resonance imaging and computed tomography along with image-processing technology that allows rapid, automated fusion of imaging modalities. In addition, stereotactic brain atlases, produced with cadaver brains sliced and oriented with respect to landmarks such as the anterior and posterior commissures (Morel et al. 1997; Schaltenbrand and Wahren 1977), can be overlaid and nonlinearly "morphed" to a particular patient's anatomical imaging data, further facilitating target selection. Routine use of intraoperative physiological mapping has been instrumental in the growth of functional neurosurgery for neurologic disease, in which all targets have been cell nuclei with characteristic physiological signatures. A number of methods of intraoperative physiological verification of the anatomical target exist: microelectrode recording, semimicroelectrode recording, and macrostimulation. Both microelectrode and semimicroelectrode recording are used to define the boundaries of a given structure on the basis of known spontaneous or evoked electrical activity of that structure and surrounding structures.

Stimulation Technique

In DBS, a brain lead 1.27 mm in diameter is implanted stereotactically with millimeter accuracy into specific brain targets. There are four platinum/iridium electrode contacts on each lead, and typically one lead is implanted on each side. The stimulating leads are connected via an extension wire to pulse generators typically placed in the chest. The devices, sometimes called "brain pacemakers," are manufactured by Medtronic (Minneapolis, MN).

The leads themselves have several independently program-mable electrode contact sites, making the anatomical extent of stimulation adjustable. Frequency, intensity, and pulse width also are programmable, within safety limits restricting the den-sity of the electrical charge induced. Chronic stimulation can be unipolar, bipolar, or multipolar because each of the electrode con-tacts can be used as an anode or cathode to provide a variety of electrical field patterns. Stimulation parameters include fre-quency ranges of 2–185 Hz, voltage range of 0–10.5 volts, and pulse widths ranging from 60 to 450 microseconds. The stimula-tors are programmed with a portable device that communicates with the implanted generator by telemetry. Stimulation can be performed continuously or intermittently and can be pro-grammed to cycle on and off during fixed time intervals. Patient programming devices allow patients to activate and deactivate the stimulator with handheld controllers and can be used to modify a subset of the stimulation parameters within given lim-its set by the treatment or investigative team.

This large potential parameter space provides both an oppor-tunity to optimize therapy and a challenge to doing so. Although it has much more anatomical precision than rTMS, DBS, like rTMS and to some extent vagus nerve stimulation, has a large number of potential combinations of stimulation parameters. De-spite this challenge of parameter optimization, stimulation can in theory be optimized for any given target to enhance a therapeutic response or to minimize adverse effects.

A major advantage of DBS compared with conventional abla-tive neurosurgery is that DBS is reversible. Although irreversible side effects of DBS implantation are possible (see the Adverse Ef-fects section of this chapter), the technique contrasts to ablative procedures, in which focal lesions are produced. Ablative proce-dures are currently in use in the care of a small number of pa-tients with intractable obsessive-compulsive disorder (OCD) and depression (Greenberg et al. 2003). Implantation of the brain lead is not intended to significantly damage brain tissue, and the stim-ulation itself can be modified or discontinued if side effects occur. The devices themselves can be removed. Removal of implantable pulse generators and connecting (extension) wires imposes little risk. Risks of removal of the brain leads, primarily hemorrhage, have not been definitively established; no published data address this issue. The risk of lead removal would be expected to be less than that of lead insertion (because the latter may require several passes). Anecdotal evidence thus far suggests that this is the case (A. Rezai, unpublished observations, August 2003).

Mechanisms of Action of Deep Brain Stimulation

The exact mechanism of action of brain stimulation remains unknown. Most likely, brain stimulation exerts its effects through a number of differing but interrelated mechanisms that come into play depending on the site of stimulation, the disease being treated, and the stimulation parameters used. Evidence supports a number of potential mechanisms. DBS at high frequencies (approximately 100 Hz or greater, as typically used clinically for movement disorders) has been proposed as inhibiting transmission by one or more of the following actions: 1) depolarization blockade, 2) synaptic fatigue, or 3) "neural jamming" (imposing a physiologically meaningless pattern of activity within the affected circuits). Any of these phenomena would in effect produce a "functional lesion," mimicking the effect of an actual therapeutic lesion procedure through a nondestructive mechanism. The parallel is inexact, however, in that the clinical effects of lesions and of DBS on movement disorders do not always correspond. There are other possible mechanisms of action, including that the stimulation does not inhibit information flow within key neural pathways but actually enhances it, reducing chaotic information processing through a phenomenon known as *stochastic resonance* (Montgomery and Baker 2000). Another important point is that the net effect of DBS on the functional state of a structure or pathway may change as distance from the electrode increases. Undoubtedly, the clinical effects of brain stimulation reflect the complex combination of inhibition and activation of cell bodies and axons and depend on the orientation of the electrode, the cytoarchitecture of the structure being stimulated, and frequency, pulse width, and duration of stimulation (McIntyre and Grill

2002). Active research in clinical and preclinical laboratories (Benabid et al. 2002; Vitek 2002) is expected to help identify which of the proposed physiological mechanisms are most relevant to the clinical effects of DBS. An additional avenue for research on the functional effects of DBS is being opened by findings that the devices are compatible with certain magnetic resonance imaging systems (Finelli et al. 2002; Rezai et al. 2002).

Adverse Effects

The complications of DBS can be separated into those related to the surgical procedure, the device and equipment, and the stimulation itself. The major risks of device implantation exist because a small amount of tissue is displaced and damage to the vasculature is possible. Thus seizure, hemorrhage, and infection are possible consequences of lead implantation. Experience with DBS for movement disorders indicates that the incidence of these adverse effects ranges from less than 1% to 3% for seizure, from 1% to 5% for hemorrhage, and from 2% to 25% for infection (DBS for Parkinson's Disease Study Group 2001; Koller et al. 1997; Oh et al. 2002; Rosenow and Mogilner, in press; Schuurman et al. 2000). Most infections are superficial and involve the implantable pulse generator pocket and the connecting wires. Cerebritis and brain abscess are extremely rare. The rate of device-related complications ranges from 5% to 15%. These complications include fracture of leads, disconnection, lead movement, and malfunction (DBS for Parkinson's Disease Study Group 2001; Koller et al. 1997; Oh et al. 2002; Rosenow et al., in press; Schuurman et al. 2000). These complications are less common with increasing surgical expertise and evolution of device technology. In addition, extremely rare but very serious side effects (including the deaths of two patients) have occurred when patients with implanted DBS systems have been exposed to therapeutic ultrasound or diathermy. Not surprisingly, when DBS is effective, battery depletion can result in reemergence of symptoms.

Adverse effects due to stimulation are the most common, but they are fully reversible with changes in stimulation technique. Many of these stimulation-related effects prove transient even without changes in parameters. Stimulation-induced effects can include paresthesias, muscle contraction, dysarthria, and diplopia. Landau and Perlmutter (1999), among others, have described effects on mood, memory, and cognition. In patients with primary neuropsychiatric illness, untoward changes in affect, anxiety, and other core symptoms (such as obsessive thoughts or compulsive urges) are a distinct possibility.

Deep Brain Stimulation for Intractable Obsessive-Compulsive Disorder

Landau and Perlmutter (1999), among others, reported that DBS produced marked affective changes in patients with movement disorders. This observation is quite intriguing in itself and suggests that DBS can modulate activity in neural circuits important in psychopathological states or, potentially, in response to treatment.

The rationale for development of DBS for OCD is similar to that for tremor and Parkinson's disease. Identification of surgical lesions with therapeutic effects in those illnesses was followed by the discovery that DBS applied to the same structures at high frequencies also had therapeutic effects. This rationale is strengthened by the fact that the thalamocortical loops targeted in Parkinson's disease parallel those most strongly implicated in OCD, although current lesion procedures target different sites for the two illnesses.

The most consistent findings in untreated obsessive-compulsive patients are increased glucose metabolism or blood flow in the medial and orbitofrontal cortex and anterior cingulate gyrus, the caudate nucleus, and to a lesser extent, the thalamus. These elevations in activity are, to varying degrees, accentuated during symptom provocation. Effective treatment with medications or behavior therapy tends to normalize activity in these same regions, which are thought to comprise circuits in which dysfunction is associated with the OCD symptoms of obsessive thoughts, compulsive actions, and anxiety (Greenberg et al. 2000; Insel 1992; Saxena and Rauch 2000). This finding suggests that use of DBS to alter activity in those circuits may have therapeutic potential.

There is thus far only one report in the literature on DBS used for a primary neuropsychiatric illness, intractable OCD. Preliminary evidence from a study of DBS of the anterior limb of the internal capsule in the care of four severely ill patients with treatment-refractory OCD has been published. In the initial case series, described by Nuttin and colleagues (1999), in Belgium, DBS lead implantation followed the trajectory of the anterior limb of the internal capsule, as in the earlier technique of thermocapsulotomy. The brief report by Nuttin et al. indicated that DBS was well tolerated and may have beneficial effects in the treatment of intractable OCD. In 2002, the effects of DBS of the subthalamic nucleus in two patients with severe Parkinson's disease who also had moderately severe OCD were reported. In that study, improvement in OCD symptoms was substantial within 2 weeks after the start of DBS (Mallet et al. 2002). In one of the two patients, OCD improvement occurred despite little change in parkinsonian symptoms.

Our collaborative group at Butler Hospital/Brown University and the Cleveland Clinic is testing the therapeutic effectiveness and safety of DBS of the anterior limb of the internal capsule in patients with intractable OCD. All candidates for the procedure undergo extensive screening and baseline assessment. This detailed evaluation assures that prospective patients have OCD as the primary diagnosis, are capable of fully informed consent, and meet operational criteria for illness severity and treatment refractoriness. Although we have observed beneficial effects similar to those reported by Nuttin et al., the study is ongoing, and no conclusions can be drawn until its completion. On the basis of our experience with an open study of gamma knife capsulotomy in a large series of patients with intractable OCD (Rasmussen et al., unpublished data, December 2003), we expect that accurate assessment of the therapeutic benefit and side-effect burden of DBS in this population will be possible only after months to more than a year of chronic stimulation.

Ethical Issues and Recommendations

DBS is now a conventional therapeutic option for intractable movement disorders. The efficacy of the procedure is well established, although questions remain about optimal stimulation targets and techniques for movement disorders. Although serious adverse events are possible, the overall side-effect burden is favorable. DBS has therefore become an attractive therapeutic option for an otherwise untreatable group of patients who experience tremendous suffering and functional impairment. That interest in DBS as a potential treatment of patients with severe neuropsychiatric illness is growing rapidly is not surprising. Such patients experience extreme distress and inability to participate in social and occupational life. As is true of movement disorders, development of modern lesion procedures as treatment of last resort of a subgroup of severely affected patients with neuropsychiatric illness (Greenberg et al. 2003) has led to identification of potential anatomical targets for DBS.

There are strong parallels between the existing application of DBS in the management of intractable neurological illness and its potential use in neuropsychiatry. There are also differences. The most salient of these arises from historical experience. Special concern over the use of neurosurgery for psychiatric illnesses is mainly the legacy of the widespread use of early destructive procedures, particularly frontal lobotomy, in the mid-twentieth century. Many patients underwent that surgery before adequate long-term safety data were obtained and without careful characterization of the primary disorder. Tragic consequences were frequent and remain a vivid reminder of the need for caution in this area.

An interdisciplinary group of collaborators has formed to systematically study the effectiveness and safety of DBS for intractable OCD. The group has recently recommended that certain requirements be met, at a minimum, for psychiatrists and neurosurgeons contemplating using DBS for psychiatric indications (OCD-DBS Collaborative Group, 2002). Several issues are worth highlighting, beginning with the strong recommendation that this work be done only as part of an investigational protocol. Initial and ongoing review must be conducted by an institutional review board (United States) or ethics committee. In the United States, there is additional review by the Food and Drug Administration, to which investigators apply for an Investigational Device Exemption to pursue this work.

Careful psychiatric assessment is an extremely important requirement. Psychiatrists must make certain that patients are selected carefully. Patients must meet operational criteria for the primary neuropsychiatric disorder under study and for the severity of that illness. It is just as important to ensure that all proven medication and cognitive/behavioral therapies have been given adequate trials and exhausted. We propose that the cases of patients who may be candidates for DBS also undergo a second level of consideration by an interdisciplinary review committee with appropriate expertise, including a bioethics perspective, that is independent from the investigative team. This research should be done at specialized academic research centers with extensive experience in the treatment of patients with the neuropsychiatric condition in question, especially intractable illness. The neurosurgical team also should have substantial experience with DBS as currently practiced.

It is extremely important that postoperative management be optimized. At the current state of the field, postoperative care can be quite time-consuming. Adequate provision must be made for patient monitoring, stimulation adjustment, and coordination of other pharmacological and behavioral therapies.

Conclusion

DBS is established therapy for movement disorders. It is an investigational treatment of other neurological conditions and of neuropsychiatric illnesses. In DBS, neuroanatomical sites deep within the brain are targeted that are proposed to be centrally involved in the pathophysiologic mechanisms of some neuropsychiatric illnesses. DBS is nonablative, offering the advantages of reversibility and adjustability. This feature may allow enhancement of therapeutic effectiveness and minimization of side effects. In preclinical and clinical studies, investigators have shown effects of DBS both locally at the stimulation target and at a distance, through actions on fibers of passage or across synapses. Although the mechanisms of action are not fully elucidated, several effects have been proposed to underlie the therapeutic effects of DBS in movement disorders and possibly in other conditions.

The mechanisms of action of DBS are the focus of active investigation in a number of clinical and preclinical laboratories. As in severe movement disorders, DBS may offer a degree of hope for patients with intractable neuropsychiatric illness. It is already clear that research intended to realize this potential will require considerable commitment of resources, energy, and time, across disciplines including psychiatry, neurosurgery, neurology, neuropsychology, bioengineering, and bioethics. These investigations should proceed cautiously.

References

Benabid AL, Benazzous A, Pollak P: Mechanisms of deep brain stimulation. Mov Disord 17 (suppl 3):S73–S74, 2002

DBS for Parkinson's Disease Study Group: Deep-brain stimulation of the subthalamic nucleus or the pars interna of the globus pallidus in Parkinson's disease. N Engl J Med 345:956–963, 2001

Deuschl G, Bain P: Deep brain stimulation for tremor [correction of trauma]: patient selection and evaluation. Mov Disord 17 (suppl 3):S102–S111, 2002

Finelli DA, Rezai AR, Ruggieri PM, et al: MR imaging-related heating of deep brain stimulation electrodes: in vitro study. AJNR Am J Neuroradiol 23:1795–1802, 2002

Greenberg BD, Murphy DL, Rasmussen SA, et al: Neuroanatomically based approaches to obsessive-compulsive disorder: neurosurgery and transcranial magnetic stimulation. Psychiatr Clin North Am 23:671–686, 2000

Greenberg BD, Price LH, Rauch SL, et al: Neurosurgery for intractable obsessive-compulsive disorder and depression: critical issues. Neurosurg Clin N Am 14:199–212, 2003

Hodaie M, Wennberg RA, Dostrovsky JO, et al: Chronic anterior thalamus stimulation for intractable epilepsy. Epilepsia 43:603–608, 2002

Insel TR: Toward a neuroanatomy of obsessive-compulsive disorder. Arch Gen Psychiatry 49:739–744, 1992

Just H, Ostergaard K: Health-related quality of life in patients with advanced Parkinson's disease treated with deep brain stimulation of the subthalamic nuclei. Mov Disord 17:539–545, 2002

Koller W, Pahwa R, Busenbark K, et al: High-frequency unilateral thalamic stimulation in the treatment of essential and parkinsonian tremor. Ann Neurol 42:292–299, 1997

Kumar K, Toth C, Nath RK, et al: Deep brain stimulation for intractable pain: a 15-year experience. Neurosurgery 40:736–746, 1997

Kumar R, Lozano AM, Sime E, et al: Comparative effects of unilateral and bilateral subthalamic nucleus deep brain stimulation. Neurology 53:561–566, 1999

Landau WM, Perlmutter JS: Transient acute depression induced by high-frequency deep-brain stimulation (letter). N Engl J Med 341:1004, 1999

Limousin P, Krack P, Pollak P et al: Electrical stimulation of the subthalamic nucleus in advanced Parkinson's disease. N Engl J Med 339: 1105–1111, 1998

Loddenkemper T, Pan A, Neme S, et al: Deep brain stimulation in epilepsy. J Clin Neurophysiol 18:514–532, 2001

Mallet L, Mesnage V, Houeto JL, et al: Compulsions, Parkinson's disease, and stimulation. Lancet 360:1302–1304, 2002

McIntyre CC, Grill WM: Extracellular stimulation of central neurons: influence of stimulus waveform and frequency on neuronal output. J Neurophysiol 88:1592–1604, 2002

Mogilner AY, Sterio D, Rezai AR, et al: Subthalamic nucleus stimulation in patients with a prior pallidotomy. J Neurosurg 96:660–665, 2002

Montgomery EB Jr, Baker KB: Mechanisms of deep brain stimulation and future technical developments. Neurol Res 22:259–266, 2000

Morel A, Magnin M, Jeanmonod D, et al: Multiarchitectonic and stereotactic atlas of the human thalamus. J Comp Neurol 387:588–630, 1997

Nuttin B, Cosyns P, Demeulemeester H, et al: Electrical stimulation in anterior limbs of internal capsules in patients with obsessive-compulsive disorder. Lancet 354:1526, 1999

OCD-DBS Collaborative Group: Deep brain stimulation for psychiatric disorders. Neurosurgery 51:519, 2002

Oh MY, Abosch A, Kim SH, et al: Long-term hardware-related complications of deep brain stimulation. Neurosurgery 50:1268–1274, 2002

Pollak P, Fraix V, Krack P, et al: Treatment results: Parkinson's disease. Mov Disord 17 (suppl 3):S75–S83, 2002

Rezai AR, Mogilner AY, Cappell J, et al: Integration of functional brain mapping in image-guided neurosurgery. Acta Neurochir Suppl 68:85–89, 1997

Rezai AR, Finelli D, Nyenhuis JA, et al: Neurostimulation systems for deep brain stimulation: in vitro evaluation of magnetic resonance imaging-related heating at 1.5 tesla. J Magn Reson Imaging 15:241–250, 2002

Rosenow JM, Mogilner AY: Deep brain stimulation for movement disorders. Neurol Res (in press)

Saxena S, Rauch SL: Functional neuroimaging and the neuroanatomy of obsessive-compulsive disorder. Psychiatr Clin North Am 23:563–586, 2000

Schaltenbrand G, Wahren W: Atlas for Stereotaxy of the Human Brain. Stuttgart, Thieme, 1977

Schiff ND, Plum F, Rezai AR, et al: Developing prosthetics to treat cognitive disabilities resulting from acquired brain injuries. Neurol Res 24:116–124, 2002

Schuurman PR, Bosch DA, Bossuyt PM, et al: A comparison of continuous thalamic stimulation and thalamotomy for suppression of severe tremor. N Engl J Med 342:461–468, 2000

Tasker RR: Deep brain stimulation is preferable to thalamotomy for tremor suppression. Surg Neurol 49:145–153, 1998

Vercueil L, Krack P, Pollak P, et al: Results of deep brain stimulation for dystonia: a critical reappraisal. Mov Disord 17 (suppl 3):S89–S93, 2002

Vingerhoets FJ, Villemure JG, Temperli P, et al: Subthalamic DBS replaces levodopa in Parkinson's disease: two-year follow-up. Neurology 58:396–401, 2002

Vitek JL: Mechanisms of deep brain stimulation: excitation or inhibition. Mov Disord 17 (suppl 3):S69–S72, 2002

Voges J, Volkmann J, Allert N, et al: Bilateral high-frequency stimulation in the subthalamic nucleus for the treatment of Parkinson disease: correlation of therapeutic effect with anatomical electrode position. J Neurosurg 96:269–279, 2002

Volkmann J, Benecke R: Deep brain stimulation for dystonia: patient selection and evaluation. Mov Disord 17 (suppl 3):S112–S115, 2002

Volkmann J, Allert N, Voges J, et al: Safety and efficacy of pallidal or subthalamic nucleus stimulation in advanced PD. Neurology 56:548–551, 2001

Yamamoto T, Katayama Y, Oshima H, et al: Deep brain stimulation therapy for a persistent vegetative state. Acta Neurochir Suppl 79:79–82, 2002

Chapter 4

Magnetic Seizure Therapy

Development of a Novel Convulsive Technique

Sarah H. Lisanby, M.D.

Electroconvulsive therapy (ECT) remains the most effective treatment of severe major depression and plays an important role in the treatment of other psychiatric disorders (American Psychiatric Association 2001). Over the 70 years since its introduction, ECT has undergone numerous revisions that have improved its safety profile, including use of general anesthesia, refinements in electrical stimulus parameters, introduction of unilateral and bifrontal electrode placement, and enhanced control of electrical dosage relative to the threshold for induction of seizure. Each advance has been accompanied by improvements in the risk/benefit ratio of this highly effective treatment. With the availability of high-power magnetic stimulators, it is now possible to perform convulsive therapy by using a magnetic stimulus rather than an electrical stimulus to induce the seizure. Magnetic fields pass through tissue without the impedance encountered by direct application of electricity, making it possible to focus the site and extent of stimulation more precisely than is possible with conventional ECT (Sackeim 1994). Magnetic seizure therapy (MST) entails use of repetitive transcranial magnetic stimulation (rTMS) to trigger a seizure from superficial cortex (Lisanby 2002).

Supported in part by National Institute of Mental Health grants K08 MH01577 and R01 MH60884, the Stanley Foundation, a Paul Beeson Physician Faculty Scholars Award from the American Federation for Aging Research, and the National Alliance for Research on Schizophrenia and Depression.

Like the other emerging brain stimulation technologies discussed in this volume, MST is investigational. Researchers in the field are just beginning to explore the potential utility of this technique in psychiatry. In this chapter I review the rationale for MST, the course of its development, and the present state of knowledge from preclinical and clinical studies concerning mechanisms of action and a possible therapeutic role in psychiatry.

Definitions and Regulatory Status

Repetitive transcranial magnetic stimulation refers to a noninvasive means of stimulating the cortex with rapidly alternating magnetic fields applied to the scalp with a portable electromagnetic coil (Barker et al. 1985). rTMS can be administered without anesthesia in an ambulatory setting with the appropriate equipment and staffing for management of seizure—the most serious known risk of rTMS. rTMS is under investigation for its therapeutic potential in a number of psychiatric and neurological disorders, including major depressive disorder, bipolar disorders, schizophrenia, anxiety disorders, epilepsy, dystonia, tic disorders, and Parkinson's disease (see Burt et al. 2002; George et al. 1999; Wassermann et al. 2001 for reviews). Apart from its still to be determined therapeutic role, rTMS has already been demonstrated to be a useful and unique tool for studying brain function in health and disease. rTMS, in combination with functional neuroimaging, can yield information about functional brain activity, connectivity, and plasticity (see, for example, Cohen et al. 1997; Lisanby et al. 2002; Paus et al. 1997). Unlike imaging, which is correlative, rTMS is a brain intervention that alters neuronal excitability in a regionally specific manner, allowing direct examination of the functional role of the stimulated cortex.

The first transcranial magnetic stimulator was introduced in 1985 (Barker et al. 1985). In the United States, rTMS devices are labeled by the Food and Drug Administration for peripheral nerve stimulation by prescription use only (i.e., under a licensed physician's supervision). Use of rTMS devices to stimulate the brain is considered investigational, requiring approval from the Food and Drug Administration (in the United States) and local institutional review board or ethics committee for each study. "Off-label" use of investigational devices is permitted in the United States under the "Practice of Medicine Provision" (Federal Food, Drug, and Cosmetic Act of 1938, Pub. L. No. 75-717) provided the device is used by a licensed physician to treat a disease or condition within a legitimate physician-patient relationship and provided there is no advertising or promotion of the off-label use. Widespread off-label use of investigational devices is generally discouraged until the body of published evidence is substantial enough to support its safety and efficacy. There is also concern that extensive off-label use may hamper enrollment in the research studies required to determine the safety and efficacy of the device.

Magnetic seizure therapy refers to the use of rTMS to induce a seizure for therapeutic purposes (Lisanby et al. 2001b). The goal of MST is to improve the tolerability of ECT through better control over the site of seizure onset and patterns of seizure spread, because these factors are thought to be major contributors to the efficacy and side effects of ECT. As currently practiced, MST is performed under general anesthesia in an ECT suite by medical personnel experienced in the conduct of ECT (Lisanby et al. 2001c). Like ECT, the MST procedure is performed once a day, three times a week, although the optimal dosing schedule has not yet been systematically studied. The device used to perform MST is a modified version of an rTMS device (Figure 4–1) that has an extended output range to overcome the anticonvulsant effects of anesthesia (Table 4–1). Like rTMS, MST is considered investigational and is currently performed only in the context of approved research studies.

Rationale for Magnetic Seizure Therapy

MST was conceived of as a means of reducing the cognitive side effects of ECT (Sackeim 1994). ECT is the most effective and rapidly acting treatment of major depressive disorders and the depressive phase of bipolar disorders (American Psychiatric Association 2001), but its use is limited by cognitive and other side effects (Lisanby et al. 2000; Squire et al. 1975). A form of con-

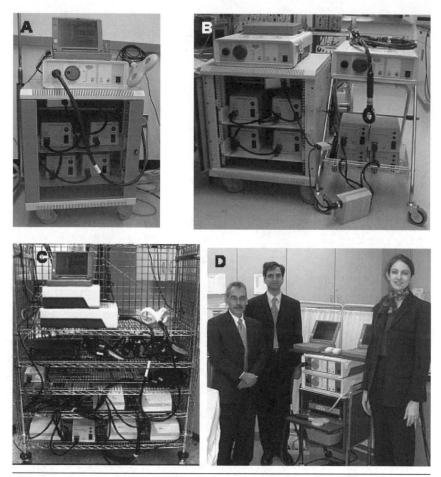

Figure 4–1. Repetitive transcranial magnetic stimulation and magnetic seizure therapy (MST) device configurations.

(A) The commercially available Super Rapid device (Magstim, Whitland, Wales), which has four booster modules and a maximum output of 25 Hz, 100%, 10 seconds, was underpowered to induce seizures under anesthesia in rats, monkeys, and humans. *(B)* The custom-modified MST device (Magstim), which has eight booster modules and a maximum output of 40 Hz, 100%, 6.3 seconds, induced seizures in monkeys under anesthesia but was underpowered for most human patients. *(C)* The current-generation MST device (Magstim), which has 16 booster modules and a maximum output of 60 Hz, 100%, 6.6 seconds, reliably induced seizures in monkeys and human patients under anesthesia but not in rodents, even without anesthesia. *(D) From left,* Drs. Harold A. Sackeim, Reza Jalinous, and Sarah Lisanby at the first clinical trial of MST treatment in the United States, November 27, 2000.

Table 4–1. Repetitive transcranial magnetic simulation (rTMS) and magnetic seizure therapy (MST) device specifications

Specification	rTMS device	8-booster MST	16-booster MST
Number of charging units (boosters)	4	8	16
Power requirements (amperes)	80	160	320
Pulse width (milliseconds)	0.2	0.5	0.5
Frequency (Hz)	25	40	60
Maximum train duration at peak frequency (seconds)	10	6.3	6.6
Seizure induction in unanesthetized rat	No	No	No
Seizure induction in anesthetized monkey	No	Yes	Yes
Seizure induction in anesthetized human	No	Limited	Yes

vulsive therapy that retains the therapeutic efficacy of ECT but reduces its side effects should substantially improve the quality of life for patients needing convulsive therapy and remove a clinically important barrier to accessing this highly effective treatment. MST is under development as a means of achieving that goal and may be viewed in the broader context of other modifications of ECT technique that have been developed over the past 70 years (Lisanby et al. 2003b).

Refinements in electrode placement and parameters of stimulation have dramatically improved the side-effect profile of ECT. For example, it has long been recognized that right unilateral ECT has fewer side effects than bilateral ECT (Squire 1977). Although substantial work has shown that response rates to right unilateral ECT tend to be lower than for bilateral ECT, it has now been demonstrated that the two electrode placements can be equally effective when right unilateral ECT is administered at sufficiently high dosages (McCall et al. 2000; Sackeim et al. 2000b). Importantly, high-dosage right unilateral ECT retains cognitive advantages relative to bilateral ECT. Thus reductions in side effects need not necessarily be linked to reduced efficacy.

Despite attempts to optimize ECT technique, the risk of amnesia remains a significant concern for patients, causing some to reject referrals to ECT and dissuading some clinicians from suggesting this important acute and maintenance treatment option. Developing an alternative for these patients demands a working knowledge of the mechanisms of action of ECT so that these can be retained and optimized, as well as an understanding of the mechanisms underlying the adverse cognitive effects so that these can be minimized. Such knowledge is central to advancing the science of ECT and to laying the groundwork for improvements in ECT technique, be they magnetic or electrical. Implicit in any attempt to improve the risk/benefit ratio of ECT is the supposition that the mechanisms underlying efficacy and side effects can be at least partially separated. Identifying these mechanisms represents a major challenge and has been the topic of an extensive body of work in the field of ECT. Clues to these mechanisms come from comparing the neurophysiological, neuroendocrine, neuroanatomical, and other effects of various forms of

ECT that differ in efficacy and side effects. Apart from the putative therapeutic role, which is yet to be determined, the development of a novel convulsive technique that differs from ECT in key neurobiological effects should be informative regarding which of the many actions of ECT are critical to efficacy and to what degree efficacy and side effects can be separated.

Double-masked, randomized trials have demonstrated powerful interactions between electrode placement and dosage in regard to the efficacy and side effects of ECT (Sackeim et al. 1993, 2000a). This observation and the finding that forms of ECT that differ in efficacy also differ in regional brain activity have been interpreted as indicating that sites of seizure onset and patterns of seizure spread are critical to determining the clinical effects of ECT. Certain changes in regional cerebral blood flow (Awata et al. 2002; Nobler et al. 1994), cerebral metabolic rate for glucose (Henry et al. 2001; Nobler et al. 2001), and electroencephalographic (EEG) measures (Sackeim et al. 1996, 2000a) correlate with the efficacy and cognitive side effects of ECT. ECT induces widespread and highly significant decreases in regional cerebral metabolism, the largest reductions occurring in bilateral superior, dorsolateral, and medial prefrontal cortices (Nobler et al. 2001). Other regions heavily involved include bilateral parietal cortex, posterior cingulate gyrus, and left medial and inferior temporal lobe. It is thought that the prefrontal changes are associated with antidepressant efficacy and that the temporal changes are related to the amnestic side effects of the treatment. In support of this notion, antidepressant response was found to be correlated with prefrontal cerebral blood flow reductions and increases in prefrontal slowing on EEG tracings (Sackeim et al. 1996). Furthermore, measures of retrograde amnesia for autobiographical memories correlated with increased left frontotemporal EEG theta power (Luber et al. 2000; Nobler et al. 2000).

It is not surprising that the effects of ECT on prefrontal circuitry appear to be central to its efficacy, considering the important role that this region plays in distributed cortical-striatal-limbic networks implicated in depression (Mayberg 1997). Blood flow and metabolism deficits in the prefrontal cortex, especially in the dorsolateral prefrontal cortex, have been widely replicated in states of depression (Baxter et al. 1989; Bench et al. 1992; Dolan et al. 1992; Mayberg 1994; Mayberg et al. 1994) and have been found to correlate with depression severity (Austin et al. 1992; Drevets et al. 1992). At least some of these changes have been reported to become altered after antidepressant response to treatment (Baxter et al. 1985, 1989; Bench et al. 1995) even if that treatment is placebo (Mayberg et al. 2002). There are clues that functional deficits in subgenual prefrontal cortex may be associated with underlying anatomical changes in this region in patients with familial depression (Drevets et al. 1997). Heterogeneity in these findings among depressed persons can be important for predicting clinical response. For example, baseline hyperactivity in rostral anterior cingulate gyrus is predictive of antidepressant response, whereas baseline hypoactivity is predictive of the opposite, suggesting that this area plays a role in mediating response (Mayberg et al. 2002). The existence of this phenomenon also suggests that baseline patterns of blood flow and metabolism in depressed persons reflect a combination of state markers, trait markers, and functional or dysfunctional compensatory processes. This finding presents an additional challenge to translating imaging findings into a focal treatment strategy.

The ability to use models of depression circuitry to develop a focal treatment and thereby to test the validity of these models is hampered by the relative spatial imprecision of ECT. Direct application of electricity through the scalp represents a physical barrier to control over the site and extent of stimulation with ECT (Sackeim et al. 1994). The impedance of the scalp and skull blocks the flow of electricity and shunts the bulk of the stimulus away from the brain. The net result is a lack of control over the site of stimulation. Variability in anatomy across individuals causes inconsistent amounts of stimulation to reach the brain and may explain in part the wide range in seizure threshold with ECT.

Although both MST and ECT induce seizures through electrical stimulation of the brain (indirectly by electromagnetic induction in the case of MST), the electrical field induced by MST is more focal than that induced by ECT (Lisanby et al. 2003c). The currents induced by ECT are radial in orientation and can pass through deep brain structures. The currents induced by MST are tangential to the surface of the brain and drop off exponentially with distance from the stimulating coil. Because magnetic fields pass through tissue unimpeded, there is greater control over the site and extent of stimulation with MST. The electrical field induced by rTMS is capable of neural depolarization at a depth of approximately 2 cm below the scalp (i.e., gray–white matter junction), so direct effects are limited to the cortex (Epstein 1990). In addition, depending principally on coil geometry, the magnetic field can be spatially targeted in cortical regions, offering further control over intracerebral current paths (Brasil-Neto et al. 1992; Maccabee et al. 1990, 1991). This enhanced control represents a way to focus the treatment in targeted cortical structures thought to mediate antidepressant response and to reduce spread to medial temporal structures implicated in the amnestic side effects of ECT.

Development of Magnetic Seizure Therapy

The idea of using rTMS to induce seizures was first raised in the field of neurology as a potential means of confirming diagnosis, localizing seizure focus, and presurgical planning in the care of epileptic patients (Dhuna et al. 1991; Hufnagel et al. 1990; Steinhoff et al. 1993). That work demonstrated that using rTMS to produce seizures on demand in epileptic patients was exceedingly difficult, especially in medicated patients. In 1993, results of studies on the safety of rTMS demonstrated that at sufficient dosages, rTMS could induce generalized seizures inadvertently in healthy human subjects who had not received medication (Pascual-Leone et al. 1993). The results of those studies prompted development of safety guidelines for limiting and individualizing rTMS dosage to avoid inadvertent seizure induction. Sackeim first proposed the idea of using rTMS to deliberately induce seizures under anesthesia as a means of improving ECT through greater control over sites of seizure onset and patterns of seizure spread (Sackeim 1994). For this application, the rTMS device would have to overcome the anticonvulsant action of the general anesthesia routinely used during ECT. Early work demonstrated that commercially available rTMS devices were underpowered for achieving that goal (Table 4–1 and Figure 4–1). Developing a device capable of reliable seizure induction under anesthesia required several years of developmental work in an animal model.

MST is at a very early stage of development. As of this writing, a worldwide total of 16 nonhuman primates and 26 human patients with major depression have received MST. Results from these preclinical and clinical studies are summarized.

Preclinical Studies With Magnetic Seizure Therapy

Nonhuman Primate Model of Magnetic Seizure Therapy and Electroconvulsive Shock

My colleagues and I obtained results that suggested nonhuman primates were the ideal animal model for MST, mostly because of their large brain size relative to other commonly used experimental animals (Lisanby et al. 2001b). We have not found it possible to induce seizures with rTMS in rodents (even in unanesthetized subjects) at high levels of stimulation (up to 60 Hz, 100% maximal stimulator output [2 tesla], 6.6-second trains, small figure-eight or round coils). This outcome likely occurred because the intensity of the electrical field induced in the brain was proportional to the size of the brain and because of the ratio between coil size and brain size (Weissman et al. 1992). Use of pediatric-sized coils in monkeys offered a practical means of more closely approximating the coil-to-brain size ratio of humans. Monkeys also were used to test the neuropathological safety of MST in the primate brain and for examination of the cognitive side effects of MST relative to electroconvulsive shock (ECS). The tests were performed with tasks for assessment of more complex aspects of cognitive function than would be possible in rodents (Moscrip et al. 2001; Moscrip et al., in press).

Results of preliminary studies indicated that standard commercially available rTMS devices (with output limits of approximately 25 Hz, 100% output, 10 seconds) could not reliably induce seizures (Lisanby et al. 2001b). Two factors had to be modified to enable seizure induction: 1) the width of the magnetic pulse had to be lengthened to approximately 0.5 milliseconds, and 2) the output frequency had to be boosted by increasing the number of charging units (Table 4–1 and Figure 4–1). We found longer pulse widths less efficient, presumably owing to a slower rise time to peak field strength. A device capable of sustaining 40 Hz, 100% output for 6.3 seconds was successful in performance, on November 18, 1998, of the first deliberate seizure induction under general anesthesia (Lisanby et al. 2001b). Generalized tonic-clonic seizures were induced with a round coil positioned on the vertex in rhesus monkeys (Figure 4–2). The anesthetic protocol was the same as for conventional ECT. Subsequent work has characterized the neurophysiological and neuroanatomical effects of MST and compared them with ECS in the monkey model (Table 4–2).

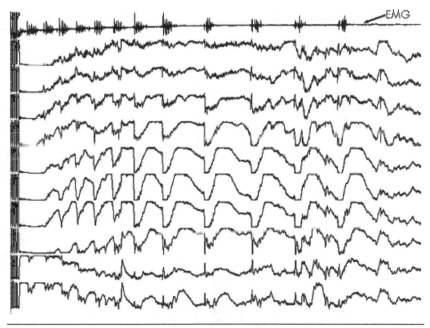

Figure 4–2. Intracerebral recordings of a seizure induced with magnetic seizure therapy in a rhesus monkey.

This seizure generalized to the motor strip and resulted in a motor convulsion as evidenced by the electromyographic (EMG) response *(top channel)*.

Source. Data from Lisanby et al. 2001b.

Table 4–2. Summary of preliminary results on magnetic seizure therapy and electroconvulsive shock in rhesus monkeys

Feature	Magnetic seizure therapy	Electroconvulsive shock
Induced electrical field		
Direction of induced currents	Tangential	Radial
Extent of stimulation	Confined to superficial cortex	Spreads to subcortical regions
Appreciable spread to hippocampus	No	Yes
Electrophysiological characteristics		
Ictal expression	Limited	Robust
Postictal suppression	Limited	Robust
Hippocampal plasticity[a]		
Mossy-fiber sprouting	Nonsignificant increase	Robust increase
Cellular proliferation	No change	Robust increase
Neuropathology[a]	No evidence of neuronal injury	No evidence of neuronal injury

[a]Anatomical studies had only four subjects per group and should be viewed as preliminary.

Spatial Distribution of the Electrical Field Induced by Magnetic Seizure Therapy

We tested the hypothesis that MST results in more focal stimulation than does ECS. Using intracerebral electrodes implanted for an extended period, we performed both procedures to measure the electrical field each induced in the brains of rhesus monkeys (Lisanby et al. 2003c). Results of these studies revealed that MST delivered sevenfold less induced charge per pulse than ECS at the site of stimulation. This disparity increased at increasing distance from the site of stimulation. MST showed negligible spread to contralateral prefrontal or ventral regions, whereas ECS induced substantial voltage at most recording sites, including ventral regions and extending to parietal and occipital cortex. Results of comparisons between MST and ECS support the hypothesis that MST is more focal and less variable in its induced electrical field than ECS. The results support the rationale for attempting seizure induction with MST as a means of limiting exposure of key brain regions to the direct effects of the induced electrical field (Figure 4–3).

Spatial Distribution of Seizures Induced by Magnetic Seizure Therapy

The greater control over the induced electrical field that can be achieved with MST is predicted to lead to greater specificity in the sites of seizure onset and patterns of seizure spread with MST compared with ECT. To compare MST and ECS in focality of seizure expression, we measured ictal power in monkeys with intracerebral electrodes (Lisanby et al. 2003c). As predicted, MST showed more differentiation in ictal expression as a function of the site of stimulation (e.g., bilateral and midline placement inducing more ictal activity in prefrontal cortex than unilateral placement) than ECS did (Figure 4–3). With ECS, seizure expression was as robust in hippocampus as in prefrontal cortex, but it was markedly less robust in hippocampus than in prefrontal cortex with MST. These data fit with the hypothesis that MST seizures are more localized to superficial cortex and show relative sparing of hippocampus. Of note, in this work we used dosages

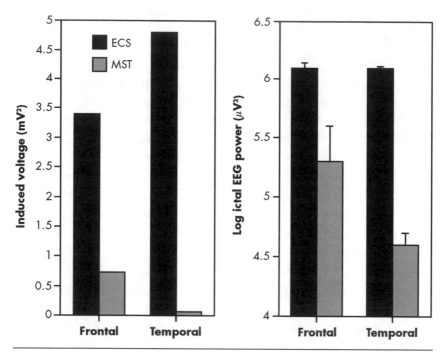

Figure 4–3.   Intracerebral recordings of the electrical field *(left)* and ictal power of the resultant seizure *(right)* induced in prefrontal and temporal cortex of rhesus monkeys with electroconvulsive shock (ECS) and magnetic seizure therapy (MST).

With ECS, electrical field strength and the intensity of seizure expression are greater in ventral and temporal regions than with MST. EEG=electroencephalographic. Error bars represent standard error.

Source.   Data from Lisanby et al. 2003c.

of MST that resulted in generalization of the seizure to the motor strip. Lower doses of MST would be expected to be even more circumscribed in their effects. Ictal expression with MST was significantly related to the distribution of the induced electrical field. As expected, this association was less strong with ECS, likely because ECS seizures generalize more robustly away from the site of initial seizure onset.

As a form of convulsive therapy with a relatively focal superficial cortical onset, MST is a means of testing whether involvement of medial and subcortical structures is necessary for efficacy and whether such involvement contributes to side effects. Two examples of involvement of deeper brain structures in which ECT and MST appear to differ are prolactin surge and hippocampal plasticity.

Prolactin Surge With Magnetic Seizure Therapy

ECT produces a characteristic and well-described acute surge in serum prolactin (Abrams et al. 1985; Fink 1986; Ohman et al. 1976; Swartz et al. 1984). Treatment factors such as electrode placement and dosage relative to threshold are major determinants of the magnitude of the prolactin surge. Although bilateral electrode placement and higher dosage relative to seizure threshold are factors that correlate with antidepressant outcome and determine the magnitude of prolactin surge, we previously reported that prolactin surge does not correlate with clinical efficacy (Lisanby et al. 1998). Prolactin surge is considered an indirect measure of the degree of diencephalic spread of the seizure. We predicted that seizures with less diencephalic spread, such as those triggered cortically with MST, would show less of a prolactin surge, indicating differential patterns of seizure spread with MST in comparison with ECT. We examined the effects of ECS and MST on serum prolactin level in rhesus monkeys (Morales et al. 2003). ECS produced a marked increase in serum prolactin in the monkeys, whereas MST caused a nonsignificant increase. This difference was consistent with the less robust seizure spread to the diencephalon with MST than with ECS. Although evidence in ECT suggests that the prolactin surge is higher with forms of ECT that carry more side effects and may be irrelevant for efficacy, the significance of the prolactin surge with MST has to be established in the context of clinical trials.

Hippocampal Plasticity in Response to Magnetic Seizure Therapy

ECS has been reported to profoundly affect two measures of hippocampal neural plasticity in rodents: mossy-fiber sprouting and neurogenesis. The former is not seen with administration of antidepressant medications and is thought to contribute to cognitive impairment in epilepsy models (Crusio et al. 1987; de Rogalski

Landrot et al. 2001; Lipp et al. 1984, 1988; Sogawa et al. 2001). The latter is seen with administration of antidepressant medications and has been hypothesized to play a role in antidepressant response (Duman et al. 2001). Contrasting the effects of MST and ECS on these two measures should be informative regarding the mechanisms underlying these effects of seizures and the feasibility of dissociating these effects through enhanced control over seizure initiation and expression.

Mossy-fiber sprouting refers to aberrant growth of collaterals of granule cell axons into the inner molecular layer of the dentate gyrus and area CA3 of the hippocampus. This sprouting is commonly seen in animal models of epilepsy (Mello et al. 1992; Represa et al. 1993, 1994) and at hippocampal resection in epileptic patients (Mathern et al. 1995). Developing a treatment devoid of a structural change in the hippocampus thought to contribute to amnestic effects would be expected to be advantageous. We reported for the first time after studies with primates that ECS, but not MST, produces significant mossy-fiber sprouting, consistent with the hypothesis that MST has less effect on medial temporal lobe structures (Lisanby et al. 2003d, 2003e).

Hippocampal neurogenesis in response to antidepressant treatment has been proposed to be a key factor mediating efficacy (Duman et al. 2001). Neurogenesis in response to seizure-induced injury, however, is thought to be related to abnormal hyperexcitability and memory disturbance associated with chronic epilepsy (Parent 2002; Parent and Lowenstein 2002; Parent et al. 1998; Scharfman et al. 2000; Scott et al. 1998). Among antidepressants, ECS is the most robust inducer of neurogenesis in rodents (Malberg et al. 2000). Because MST is more confined to superficial cortex, the effects of MST on neurogenesis should shed light on the roles of the induced electrical field and the seizure itself in this effect. Because ECS is both a seizure model and an antidepressant, the role of neurogenesis in response to ECS may be complex. Critical studies in which the neurogenesis response to ECS is blocked and the resultant effect on antidepressant action is examined have not yet been performed. A confounder of such blocking strategies is that some pharmacological agents that block neurogenesis may exert other undesirable effects. A form of convulsive therapy devoid of effects on neurogenesis by virtue of being confined to superficial cortex should provide useful information about the functional role of neurogenesis in response to seizures.

As in the results with mossy-fiber sprouting, ECS increased cellular proliferation in monkeys, whereas MST did not (Lisanby et al. 2003d, 2003e). Results of these preliminary studies suggested that merely inducing a seizure is insufficient to alter measures of hippocampal plasticity and that the spatial distribution of the induced electrical field or the pattern of seizure propagation may be critical to these effects. The clinical significance of these differences between MST and ECS has to be determined in the context of a controlled clinical trial. If MST is found to have clinical efficacy, the role of hippocampal plasticity in antidepressant action would be called into question. On the other hand, the finding that MST is ineffective in the clinical setting would support the view that an effect on hippocampal plasticity is important for the antidepressant action of seizures. A limitation of this work was that it was performed at only moderately suprathreshold levels (2.5 times seizure threshold) with a nonfocal round coil positioned on the vertex. The effects of focal prefrontal MST at more robust suprathreshold dosages, which would be expected to be closer to optimal for efficacy, are not known but are under study.

Neuropathological Studies of the Safety of Long-Term Magnetic Seizure Therapy

MST exposes the brain to magnetic fields as well as to induced electrical fields. The safety profile of magnetic field exposure is well documented by the extensive safety record of magnetic resonance imaging at field strengths of 1.5–2 tesla (and higher). The evidence presented above under "Development of Magnetic Seizure Therapy" indicates that the magnitude and distribution of the electrical fields induced in the brain by MST are substantially lower and more circumscribed than those induced with ECT and that the charge density delivered with ECT is well below levels associated with neuropathological damage (Agnew et al. 1987). Therefore MST would be expected to be as safe as or safer than ECT.

To test that hypothesis, we examined the brains of 12 rhesus monkeys randomly assigned to 6 weeks of daily treatment with MST or ECS at 2.5 times seizure threshold (Dwork et al., in press). We found complete absence of acute or remote neuropathological lesions associated with ECS or MST in this primate model, which closely mimicked clinical conditions of ECT. This work also represented the first investigation, to our knowledge, of the safety of ECS in nonhuman primates by use of modern neuropathological techniques and randomized, sham-controlled, and masked evaluation. Previous reports of neuronal loss or shrinkage with ECS were confounded by possible hypoxic effects of uncontrolled seizures and by artifacts from handling of the unfixed brain (Devanand et al. 1994). These confounders were avoided in this study by the use of general anesthesia during seizures and thorough perfusion with formalin before removal of the brain. In addition to their significance regarding the safety of MST, these data represent the most extensive exposure to rTMS in any organism and are likewise reassuring regarding the safety of subconvulsive levels of rTMS. Parenthetically, the first cohort of monkeys to receive MST, which were not part of the neuropathological studies, showed no evidence of long-term or delayed-onset detrimental behavioral effects of MST (or ECS) after nearly 5 years of follow-up study.

Clinical Trials With Magnetic Seizure Therapy

Initial Testing of Magnetic Seizure Therapy With a Human Subject

The first human to receive MST was a 20-year-old woman with medication-resistant major depressive disorder (Lisanby et al. 2001c). Treatment was rendered in the context of an institutional review board–approved case study on May 1, 2000 (Figure 4–4). This proof-of-concept case study represented my collaboration with Dr. Harold A. Sackeim of the Department of Biological Psychiatry, New York State Psychiatric Institute/Columbia University, and Drs. Thomas Schlaepfer and Hans-Ulrich Fisch of the

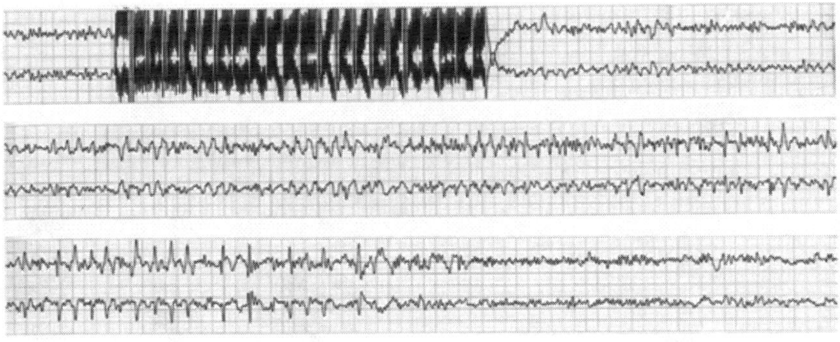

Figure 4–4. Scalp electroencephalographic recording of the first patient to receive magnetic seizure therapy (MST), Bern, Switzerland.

Dark region at beginning of tracing represents magnetic artifact resulting from current induced in the recording leads during application of MST.

Source. Lisanby et al. 2001c.

Psychiatric Neuroimaging Group, Department of Psychiatry, University Hospital Bern, Switzerland. After four MST sessions, the patient experienced a 50% decrease in score on the Hamilton Rating Scale for Depression. The treatments were well tolerated with no significant side effects.

Randomized Trial of the Acute Side Effects of Magnetic Seizure Therapy and Electroconvulsive Therapy

After the initial case demonstrated feasibility, clinical testing with MST in the United States began on November 27, 2000, with a double-masked, randomized, within-subject trial contrasting MST to ECT in regard to acute cognitive side effects and electrophysiological characteristics (Lisanby et al. 2001a, 2003a). Ten patients received a course of convulsive therapy in which two of the first four interventions were MST and the remaining treatments were conventional ECT. MST sessions were well tolerated, causing fewer subjective side effects than ECT (Figure 4–5) and faster recovery of orientation, a measure that correlates with long-term retrograde amnesia (Sobin et al. 1995). Masked neuropsychological assessment revealed largely consistent cognitive advantages of MST relative to ECT, supporting the role of current pathways

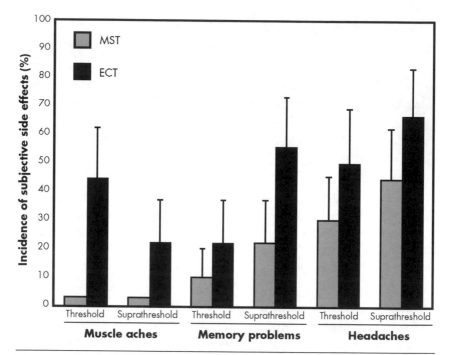

Figure 4–5. Incidence of subjective side effects reported after threshold and suprathreshold magnetic seizure therapy (MST) and electroconvulsive therapy (ECT) in 10 patients.

There was a main effect of condition: $F_{(1,8)}$=8.0, P<0.02 for muscle aches; $F_{(1,8)}$=6.4, P<0.04 for subjective memory problems; and $F_{(1,7)}$=11.67, P<0.01 for headache. Error bars represent standard error.

Source. Data from Lisanby et al. 2001a, 2003a.

and patterns of seizure expression in determining the effects of convulsive therapy. The cognitive domains in which ECT showed greater impairment than MST were generally those served at least partly by temporal lobe structures (i.e., memory for recent events, new list learning, and category fluency). This observation was consistent with the hypothesis that MST would have less effect on temporal lobe structures (Lezak 1995; Pihlajamaki et al. 2000). In contrast, tasks more heavily dependent on prefrontal lobe function did not show differences between MST and ECT (e.g., memory for temporal order and verbal fluency for letters). This observation was consistent with the view that MST would retain effects on prefrontal structures important for efficacy (Cabeza et al. 1997; Janowsky et al. 1989; Spreen and Strauss 1998). These differential neuropsychological effects provide support for the regional physiological differences between MST and ECS found with intracerebral recordings.

Marked differences in the nature of the seizures induced by ECT and MST were seen even in comparisons of seizures that generalized to the motor strip. Compared with ECT, MST seizures had shorter duration, lower ictal EEG amplitude, and less postictal suppression (Lisanby et al. 2003a). It will be important to determine whether these electrophysiological differences have clinical significance, either positive or negative. Although some of these measures are weakly correlated with the efficacy of ECT (Folkerts 1996; Krystal et al. 1995; Nobler et al. 1993; Suppes et al. 1996), recent results have called this relationship into question. Nobler et al. (2000) found only weak relations between seizure expression and clinical outcome. Results of ongoing study indicate ultrabrief-pulse right unilateral ECT lacks some EEG characteristics formerly thought to be markers of effective treatment (Sackeim et al. 2001). Ultrabrief-pulse right unilateral ECT has less robust postictal suppression than conventional forms of ECT, yet, administered at an adequate dosage relative to seizure threshold, it was as effective as conventional bilateral ECT. These results suggest that our understanding of the markers of effective treatment will evolve as novel forms of convulsive therapy are developed and tested.

Antidepressant Efficacy of Magnetic Seizure Therapy

The antidepressant efficacy of MST is not yet known. My colleagues and I are in the midst of a randomized, double-masked, two-center clinical trial comparing two forms of MST in regard to antidepressant efficacy and side effects to inform the design of a subsequent masked comparison with ECT. This study represents a collaboration between our center and Drs. Mustafa Husain and A. John Rush of the University of Texas Southwestern Medical Center. Parallel work is under way with Dr. Thomas Schlaepfer in Bern, Switzerland. The two forms of MST under examination are stimulation with the nonfocal cap coil positioned on vertex and stimulation with the focal double cone coil positioned on prefrontal cortex. To date, 20 medication-resistant patients with a major depressive episode (unipolar or bipolar) have enrolled. Extensive neuropsychological testing is under way, and patients are being observed for 6 months for evaluation for persistence of any clinical benefits or side effects. Results of this study will provide preliminary evidence for or against the antidepressant activity of MST. The comparison between the two coil types should inform selection of optimal coil type in subsequent trials comparing MST with ECT. When more experience has been gained with optimizing delivery of MST, it will be necessary to compare MST with conventional antidepressant treatments in randomized clinical trials to establish efficacy.

Current Device Limitations and Future Directions

Although the current MST device was adequate for suprathreshold stimulation in monkeys, results with human subjects indicated the device is likely underpowered for clinical applications. Forty-three percent of patients in studies to date had a seizure threshold at the maximal output of the device. No patient could be treated at 6 times threshold, a dosage that increases the efficacy of right unilateral ECT (McCall et al. 2000; Sackeim et al. 2000b) Furthermore, it has not yet been possible to induce a seizure in anesthetized patients with a focal coil positioned over the prefrontal cortex. This lack of success probably has occurred because focal coils stimulate a smaller region of cortex and induce less current than nonfocal coils, and the seizure threshold of prefrontal cortex is higher than that of other superficial cortical areas, such as primary motor cortex (Ojemann 1993). No seizures have been successfully induced in anesthetized humans with a figure-eight coil (the most focal of the available coils) over the prefrontal cortex, even at the maximal output of the stimulator. Likewise, the moderately focal double cone coil did not induce a seizure over midline prefrontal cortex in seven of nine attempts at maximal output. Accentuating the problems of limited device output, MST threshold increases throughout the treatment course, as it does also in ECT. Monkeys had an increase of 31.7%±24.6% ($t=2.8$, df=3, $P<0.03$), and patients had an increase of 66.7%±33.3% ($t=2.3$, df=9, $P<0.05$). All patients whose threshold was not at the maximal output of the stimulator at baseline had an increase in seizure threshold after the MST course. This finding suggested that MST and ECT share anticonvulsant activity, a characteristic some experts hypothesize is important to the antidepressant activity of ECT (Sackeim 1999).

If the relationship between dosage above threshold and efficacy for ECT pertains to MST, the available data from studies with humans and monkeys indicate that the current-generation MST device is incapable of providing stimulation at an adequate percentage relative to seizure threshold to maximize antidepressant efficacy. The next steps in the development of MST will involve further coil and device modifications to enable focal seizure induction in targeted prefrontal regions, better control of coil heating and noise (both of which are accentuated with MST relative to rTMS because of the higher output levels), improved ease of use by decreasing the number of power inlets required (currently 16 separate 20-ampere-rated circuits), and improved reliability of device operation. Device modifications are currently under development and being piloted in an attempt to achieve these goals.

Conclusion

MST is under development as a means of lowering the side-effect burden of ECT and thereby improving the quality of life for severely ill patients with major depression and other disorders for which ECT is at present the only treatment. MST is the most recent variation in a long history of modifications to ECT technique, yet it remains at a very early stage of development. The ultimate clinical role of MST is unknown. The evidence to date, although preliminary, supports the safety of MST and suggests its acute side-effect profile is more benign than that of ECT. Because seizures are highly effective in treating major depression, whether the seizures are induced electrically or chemically, the expectation would be that seizures triggered magnetically would follow suit. However, work over the past few decades has shown that as a function of their means of induction, ECT-induced seizures differ in efficacy and side effects. Thus it will be necessary to rigorously test the clinical efficacy of MST in the context of controlled clinical trials. Likewise, it will be important to systematically examine the parameters of stimulation with MST to determine whether and how they interact in determining efficacy and side effects. Such dose-finding work is a necessary step before randomized comparisons with ECT and should prevent premature abandonment of this new technique as the result of underdosing. If the dose-response relationships seen with ECT pertain to MST, device modifications to increase output will be necessary to optimize the efficacy of MST.

Should results of future randomized trials show that MST as it is currently being practiced is effective, it would be of great interest to scale back the parameters to determine the minimally effective dosage for further enhancement of the tolerability of the treatment. All developmental work to date has been performed with seizures that generalize to the motor strip, resulting in motor convulsions. It would be valuable to know whether focal seizures that do not generalize are effective, eliminating the need for muscular paralysis during treatment and significantly simplifying the procedure. The ultimate clinical role of MST will depend on its efficacy–side effect tradeoff. If MST is found to be more tolerable than ECT but less effective than ECT, it may still have a clinical role if its efficacy has advantages relative to medication. Another potential role of MST may be relapse prevention after ECT, on the theory that its improved tolerability will enhance compliance with short- and long-term maintenance schedules. However, the efficacy of MST in relapse prevention has not yet been examined.

Like rTMS, MST may have value as a means of probing the underlying mechanisms of antidepressant action, quite independent of its potential therapeutic role. For example, differences between ECT and MST along neurobiological variables may be informative regarding the mechanisms of action of seizures and their effect on mood networks. The finding that seizures of cortical origin that do not spread to the diencephalon or hippocampus are clinically effective would have implications for our understanding of the action of ECT. This finding also would provide the opportunity to test whether mossy-fiber sprouting and neu-rogenesis are central to antidepressant action (or cognitive side effects) without the confounding effect of pharmacological strat-egies that block these processes. It has been theorized that pre-frontal seizures should enhance efficacy and reduce side effects, but with ECT there is limited control over generalization of sei-zures for selective testing of the role of prefrontal involvement. With MST, the efficacy and side effects of more circumscribed prefrontal seizures compared with those triggered from other cortical regions could help answer this question.

Subsequent clinical studies of MST must address the many as yet unanswered questions regarding clinical efficacy (both acute response and persistence of effects) relative to ECT and antide-pressant medications, parameters of stimulation (including coil type, coil placement, and dosage) and treatment schedule (inter-val between treatments, number of treatments, and continuation and maintenance schedule) to optimize its efficacy. These chal-lenges facing MST are similar to those facing the other novel brain stimulation techniques in psychiatry—demonstrating effi-cacy and defining their ultimate role in clinical practice.

References

Abrams R, Swartz CM: Electroconvulsive therapy and prolactin release: effects of stimulus parameters. Convuls Ther 1:115–119, 1985

Agnew WF, McCreery DB: Considerations for safety in the use of ex-tracranial stimulation for motor evoked potentials. Neurosurgery 20:143–147, 1987

American Psychiatric Association: The Practice of Electroconvulsive Therapy: Recommendations for Treatment, Training and Privileging. A Task Force Report of the American Psychiatric Association, 2nd Edition. Washington, DC, American Psychiatric Association, 2001

Austin MP, Dougall N, Ross M, et al: Single photon emission tomogra-phy with 99mTc-exametazime in major depression and the pattern of brain activity underlying the psychotic/neurotic continuum. J Affect Disord 26:31–43, 1992

Awata S, Konno M, Kawashima R, et al: Changes in regional cerebral blood flow abnormalities in late-life depression following response to electroconvulsive therapy. Psychiatry Clin Neurosci 56:31–40, 2002

Barker AT, Jalinous R, Freeston IL: Non-invasive magnetic stimulation of human motor cortex. Lancet 1:1106–1107, 1985

Baxter LR Jr, Phelps ME, Mazziotta JC, et al: Cerebral metabolic rates for glucose in mood disorders: studies with positron emission tomography and fluorodeoxyglucose F 18. Arch Gen Psychiatry 42:441–447, 1985

Baxter LR Jr, Schwartz JM, Phelps ME, et al: Reduction of prefrontal cortex glucose metabolism common to three types of depression. Arch Gen Psychiatry 46:243–250, 1989

Bench CJ, Friston KJ, Brown RG, et al: The anatomy of melancholia: focal abnormalities of cerebral blood flow in major depression. Psychol Med 22:607–615, 1992

Bench CJ, Frackowiak RS, Dolan RJ: Changes in regional cerebral blood flow on recovery from depression. Psychol Med 25:247–261, 1995

Brasil-Neto JP, Cohen LG, Panizza M, et al: Optimal focal transcranial magnetic activation of the human motor cortex: effects of coil orientation, shape of the induced current pulse, and stimulus intensity. J Clin Neurophysiol 9:132–136, 1992

Burt T, Lisanby SH, Sackeim HA: Neuropsychiatric applications of transcranial magnetic stimulation: a meta-analysis. Int J Neuropsychopharmacol 5:73–103, 2002

Cabeza R, Mangels J, Nyberg L, et al: Brain regions differentially involved in remembering what and when: a PET study. Neuron 19:863–870, 1997

Cohen LG, Celnik P, Pascual-Leone A, et al: Functional relevance of cross-modal plasticity in blind humans. Nature 389:180–183, 1997

Crusio WE, Schwegler H, Lipp HP: Radial-maze performance and structural variation of the hippocampus in mice: a correlation with mossy fibre distribution. Brain Res 425:182–185, 1987

de Rogalski Landrot I, Minokoshi M, Silveira DC, et al: Recurrent neonatal seizures: relationship of pathology to the electroencephalogram and cognition. Brain Res Dev Brain Res 129:27–38, 2001

Devanand DP, Dwork AJ, Hutchinson ER, et al: Does ECT alter brain structure? Am J Psychiatry 151:957–970, 1994

Dhuna A, Gates J, Pascual-Leone A: Transcranial magnetic stimulation in patients with epilepsy. Neurology 41:1067–1071, 1991

Dolan RJ, Bench CJ, Brown RG, et al: Regional cerebral blood flow abnormalities in depressed patients with cognitive impairment. J Neurol Neurosurg Psychiatry 55:768–773, 1992

Drevets WC, Videen TO, Price JL, et al: A functional anatomical study of unipolar depression. J Neurosci 12:3628–3641, 1992

Drevets WC, Price JL, Simpson JR Jr, et al: Subgenual prefrontal cortex abnormalities in mood disorders. Nature 386:824–827, 1997

Duman RS, Nakagawa S, Malberg J: Regulation of adult neurogenesis by antidepressant treatment. Neuropsychopharmacology 25:836–844, 2001

Dwork AJ, Arango V, Underwood M, et al: Absence of histological lesions in primate models of electroconvulsive therapy (ECT) and magnetic seizure therapy (MST). Am J Psychiatry (in press)

Epstein CM: Localizing the site of magnetic brain stimulation in humans. Neurology 40:666–670, 1990

Federal Food, Drug, and Cosmetic Act of 1938, Pub. L. No. 75-717, sec 906, 52 Stat. 1040 codified as amended at 21 U.S.C. §321(h) 1994

Fink M: Neuroendocrine predictors of electroconvulsive therapy outcome: dexamethasone suppression test and prolactin. Ann N Y Acad Sci 462:30–36, 1986

Folkerts H: The ictal electroencephalogram as a marker for the efficacy of electroconvulsive therapy. Eur Arch Psychiatry Clin Neurosci 246:155–164, 1996

George MS, Lisanby SH, Sackeim HA: Transcranial magnetic stimulation: applications in neuropsychiatry. Arch Gen Psychiatry 56:300–311, 1999

Henry ME, Schmidt ME, Matochik JA, et al: The effects of ECT on brain glucose: a pilot FDG PET study. J ECT 17:33–40, 2001

Hufnagel A, Elger CE, Durwen HF, et al: Activation of the epileptic focus by transcranial magnetic stimulation of the human brain. Ann Neurol 27:49–60, 1990

Janowsky JS, Shimamura AP, Squire LR: Source memory impairment in patients with frontal lobe lesions. Neuropsychologia 27:1043–1056, 1989

Krystal AD, Weiner RD, Coffey CE: The ictal EEG as a marker of adequate stimulus intensity with unilateral ECT. J Neuropsychiatry Clin Neurosci 7:295–303, 1995

Lezak MD: Neuropsychological Assessment, 3rd Edition. New York, Oxford University Press, 1995

Lipp HP, Schwegler H, Driscoll P: Postnatal modification of hippocampal circuitry alters avoidance learning in adult rats. Science 225:80–82, 1984

Lipp HP, Schwegler H, Heimrich B, et al: Infrapyramidal mossy fibers and two-way avoidance learning: developmental modification of hippocampal circuitry and adult behavior of rats and mice. J Neurosci 8:1905–1921, 1988

Lisanby SH: Update on magnetic seizure therapy (MST): a novel form of convulsive therapy. J ECT 18:182–188, 2002

Lisanby SH, Devanand DP, Prudic J, et al: Prolactin response to electro-convulsive therapy: effects of electrode placement and stimulus dosage. Biol Psychiatry 43:146–155, 1998

Lisanby SH, Maddox JH, Prudic J, et al: The effects of electroconvulsive therapy on memory of autobiographical and public events. Arch Gen Psychiatry 57:581–590, 2000

Lisanby SH, Luber B, Barroilhet L, et al: Magnetic seizure therapy (MST): acute cognitive effects of MST compared with ECT (abstract). J ECT 17:77, 2001a

Lisanby SH, Luber B, Finck AD, et al: Deliberate seizure induction with repetitive transcranial magnetic stimulation. Arch Gen Psychiatry 58:199–200, 2001b

Lisanby SH, Schlaepfer TE, Fisch H-U, et al: Magnetic seizure induction for the treatment of major depression. Arch Gen Psychiatry 58:303–305, 2001c

Lisanby SH, Kinnunen LH, Crupain MJ: Applications of TMS to therapy in psychiatry. J Clin Neurophysiol 19:344–360, 2002

Lisanby SH, Luber B, Schlaepfer TE, et al: Safety and feasibility of magnetic seizure therapy (MST) in major depression: randomized within-subject comparison with electroconvulsive therapy. Neuropsychopharmacology 28:1852–1865, 2003a

Lisanby SH, Morales O, Payne N, et al: New developments in electro-convulsive therapy and magnetic seizure therapy. CNS Spectr 8:529–536, 2003b

Lisanby SH, Moscrip T, Morales O, et al: Neurophysiological characteristics of magnetic seizure therapy (MST) in nonhuman primates. Clin Neurophysiol 56 (suppl):81–99, 2003c

Lisanby SH, Sackeim HA, Dwork A, et al: Effects of electrically and magnetically induced seizures on synaptic remodeling and mossy fiber sprouting in the primate hippocampus (abstract). J ECT 19:57A–58A, 2003d

Lisanby SH, Sackeim HA, Dwork A, et al: Effects of electroconvulsive shock and magnetic seizure therapy on mossy fiber sprouting and cellular proliferation in the primate hippocampus. Biol Psychiatry 53 (suppl):173S, 2003e

Luber B, Nobler MS, Moeller JR, et al: Quantitative EEG during seizures induced by electroconvulsive therapy: relations to treatment modality and clinical features, II: topographic analyses. J ECT 16:229–243, 2000

Maccabee PJ, Eberle L, Amassian VE, et al: Spatial distribution of the electric field induced in volume by round and figure "8" magnetic coils: relevance to activation of sensory nerve fibers. Electroencephalogr Clin Neurophysiol 76:131–141, 1990

Maccabee PJ, Amassian VE, Eberle LP, et al: Measurement of the electric field induced in inhomogeneous volume conductors by magnetic coils: application to human spinal neurogeometry. Electroencephalogr Clin Neurophysiol 81:224–237, 1991

Malberg JE, Eisch AJ, Nestler EJ, et al: Chronic antidepressant treatment increases neurogenesis in adult rat hippocampus. J Neurosci 20:9104–9110, 2000

Mathern GW, Pretorius JK, Babb TL: Quantified patterns of mossy fiber sprouting and neuron densities in hippocampal and lesional seizures. J Neurosurg 82:211–219, 1995

Mayberg HS: Frontal lobe dysfunction in secondary depression. J Neuropsychiatry Clin Neurosci 6:428–442, 1994

Mayberg HS: Limbic-cortical dysregulation: a proposed model of depression. J Neuropsychiatry Clin Neurosci 9:471–481, 1997

Mayberg HS, Lewis PJ, Regenold W, et al: Paralimbic hypoperfusion in unipolar depression. J Nucl Med 35:929–934, 1994

Mayberg HS, Silva JA, Brannan SK, et al: The functional neuroanatomy of the placebo effect. Am J Psychiatry 159:728–737, 2002

McCall WV, Reboussin DM, Weiner RD, et al: Titrated moderately suprathreshold vs fixed high-dose right unilateral electroconvulsive therapy: acute antidepressant and cognitive effects. Arch Gen Psychiatry 57:438–444, 2000

Mello LE, Cavalheiro EA, Tan AM, et al: Granule cell dispersion in relation to mossy fiber sprouting, hippocampal cell loss, silent period and seizure frequency in the pilocarpine model of epilepsy Epilepsy Res Suppl 9:51–59, 1992

Morales O, Luber B, Kwon E, et al: Prolactin response to convulsive therapy: magnetic seizure therapy (MST) versus electroconvulsive shock (ECS) in nonhuman primates (abstract). J ECT 19:58A, 2003

Moscrip TD, Terrace HS, Sackeim HA, et al: The cognitive effects of ECS and MST in rhesus monkeys. Paper presented at the 31st Annual Meeting of the Society for Neuroscience, San Diego, CA, November 10–15, 2001. Abstract available at: http://sfn.scholarone.com/itin2001/main.html?new_page_id=126&abstract_id=11974& is_tech=0. Accessed October 29, 2003

Moscrip TD, Terrace HS, Sackeim HA, et al: A primate model of the anterograde and retrograde amnesia produced by convulsive treatment. J ECT (in press)

Nobler MS, Sackeim HA, Solomou M, et al: EEG manifestations during ECT: effects of electrode placement and stimulus intensity. Biol Psychiatry 34:321–330, 1993

Nobler MS, Sackeim HA, Prohovnik I, et al: Regional cerebral blood flow in mood disorders, III: treatment and clinical response. Arch Gen Psychiatry 51:884–897, 1994

Nobler MS, Luber B, Moeller JR, et al: Quantitative EEG during seizures induced by electroconvulsive therapy: relations to treatment modality and clinical features, I: global analyses. J ECT 16:211–228, 2000

Nobler MS, Oquendo MA, Kegeles LS, et al: Decreased regional brain metabolism after ECT. Am J Psychiatry 158:305–308, 2001

Ohman R, Walinder J, Balldin J, et al: Prolactin response to electroconvulsive therapy. Lancet 2:936–937, 1976

Ojemann GA: Functional mapping of cortical language areas in adults: intraoperative approaches, in Electrical and Magnetic Stimulation of the Brain and Spinal Cord. Edited by Devinsky BD. New York, Raven, 1993, pp 155–163

Parent JM: The role of seizure-induced neurogenesis in epileptogenesis and brain repair. Epilepsy Res 50:179–189, 2002

Parent JM, Lowenstein DH: Seizure-induced neurogenesis: are more new neurons good for an adult brain? Prog Brain Res 135:121–131, 2002

Parent JM, Janumpalli S, McNamara JO, et al: Increased dentate granule cell neurogenesis following amygdala kindling in the adult rat. Neurosci Lett 247:9–12, 1998

Pascual-Leone A, Houser CM, Reese K, et al: Safety of rapid-rate transcranial magnetic stimulation in normal volunteers. Electroencephalogr Clin Neurophysiol 89:120–130, 1993

Paus T, Jech R, Thompson CJ, et al: Transcranial magnetic stimulation during positron emission tomography: a new method for studying connectivity of the human cerebral cortex. J Neurosci 17:3178–3184, 1997

Pihlajamaki M, Tanila H, Hanninen T, et al: Verbal fluency activates the left medial temporal lobe: a functional magnetic resonance imaging study. Ann Neurol 47:470–476, 2000

Represa A, Jorquera I, Le Gal La Salle G, et al: Epilepsy induced collateral sprouting of hippocampal mossy fibers: does it induce the development of ectopic synapses with granule cell dendrites? Hippocampus 3:257–268, 1993

Represa A, Niquet J, Pollard H, et al: From seizures to neo-synaptogenesis: intrinsic and extrinsic determinants of mossy fiber sprouting in the adult hippocampus. Hippocampus 4:270–274, 1994

Sackeim HA: Magnetic stimulation therapy and ECT. Convuls Ther 10:255–258, 1994

Sackeim HA: The anticonvulsant hypothesis of the mechanisms of action of ECT: current status. J ECT 15:5–26, 1999

Sackeim HA, Prudic J, Devanand DP, et al: Effects of stimulus intensity and electrode placement on the efficacy and cognitive effects of electroconvulsive therapy. N Engl J Med 328:839–846, 1993

Sackeim HA, Long J, Luber B, et al: Physical properties and quantification of the ECT stimulus, I: basic principles. Convuls Ther 10:93–123, 1994

Sackeim HA, Luber B, Katzman GP, et al: The effects of electroconvulsive therapy on quantitative electroencephalograms: relationship to clinical outcome. Arch Gen Psychiatry 53:814–824, 1996

Sackeim HA, Luber B, Moeller JR, et al: Electrophysiological correlates of the adverse cognitive effects of electroconvulsive therapy. J ECT 16:110–120, 2000a

Sackeim HA, Prudic J, Devanand DP, et al: A prospective, randomized, double-blind comparison of bilateral and right unilateral electroconvulsive therapy at different stimulus intensities. Arch Gen Psychiatry 57:425–434, 2000b

Sackeim IIA, Prudic J, Nobler MS, et al: Ultra-brief pulse ECT and the affective and cognitive consequences of ECT (abstract). J ECT 17:77, 2001

Scharfman HE, Goodman JH, Sollas AL: Granule-like neurons at the hilar/CA3 border after status epilepticus and their synchrony with area CA3 pyramidal cells: functional implications of seizure-induced neurogenesis. J Neurosci 20:6144–6158, 2000

Scott BW, Wang S, Burnham WM, et al: Kindling-induced neurogenesis in the dentate gyrus of the rat. Neurosci Lett 248:73–76, 1998

Sobin C, Sackeim HA, Prudic J, et al: Predictors of retrograde amnesia following ECT. Am J Psychiatry 152:995–1001, 1995

Sogawa Y, Monokoshi M, Silveira DC, et al: Timing of cognitive deficits following neonatal seizures: relationship to histological changes in the hippocampus. Brain Res Dev Brain Res 131:73–83, 2001

Spreen O, Strauss E: A Compendium of Neuropsychological Tests: Administration, Norms, and Commentary. New York, Oxford University Press, 1998

Squire LR: ECT and memory loss. Am J Psychiatry 134:997–1001, 1977

Squire LR, Slater PC, Chace PM: Retrograde amnesia: temporal gradient in very long term memory following electroconvulsive therapy. Science 187:77–79, 1975

Steinhoff BJ, Stodieck SR, Zivcec Z, et al: Transcranial magnetic stimulation (TMS) of the brain in patients with mesiotemporal epileptic foci. Clin Electroencephalogr 24:1–5, 1993

Suppes T, Webb A, Carmody T, et al: Is postictal electrical silence a predictor of response to electroconvulsive therapy? J Affect Disord 41:55–58, 1996

Swartz C, Abrams R: Prolactin levels after bilateral and unilateral ECT. Br J Psychiatry 144:643–645, 1984

Wassermann EM, Lisanby SH: Therapeutic application of repetitive transcranial magnetic stimulation: a review. Clin Neurophysiology 112:1367–1377, 2001

Weissman JD, Epstein CM, Davey KR: Magnetic brain stimulation and brain size: relevance to animal studies. Electroencephalogr Clin Neurophysiol 85:215–219, 1992

Chapter 5

Vagus Nerve Stimulation

Harold A. Sackeim, Ph.D.

Brain Stimulation in Psychiatry

Of the new brain stimulation techniques used to treat psychiatric disorders, vagus nerve stimulation (VNS) is the least intuitively understandable. To place VNS in the context of these emerging modalities before reviewing the current status of research on VNS, I briefly describe other strategies for stimulating the brain. Magnetic seizure therapy (MST) is a form of convulsive therapy that substitutes a magnetic stimulus for the electrical stimulus used in electroconvulsive therapy (ECT) (Lisanby et al. 2001; Sackeim 1994). Because the magnetic stimulus is unimpeded by the scalp and skull, there is considerable control over the amount and spatial distribution of the current induced in brain tissue (Thielscher and Kammer 2002). Although MST promises greater precision than ECT regarding where in the brain seizures are initiated and the dosage or intensity of stimulation in neural tissue, there is no reason to expect the mechanisms underlying the therapeutic and adverse effects of MST to differ from those of ECT (Lisanby et al. 2003). Both the efficacy and the cognitive side effects of ECT are strongly determined by current paths (that is, by where in the brain the stimulation occurs) and the current density within those paths (determined by electrical dosage) (Sackeim et

This work was partially supported by National Institute of Mental Health grants MH35636, MH60884, MH61609, and MH63435. Dr. Sackeim has received research support from and serves as a consultant to various pharmaceutical companies and manufacturers of electroconvulsive therapy and transcranial magnetic stimulation devices. In particular, he has received research funding from and has served as a consultant to Cyberonics, Inc., in its program on vagus nerve stimulation for treatment-resistant depression.

al. 1993, 2000b). Once devices are developed that are capable of reliably inducing sufficient current density, MST will take advantage of this knowledge, targeting as sites of seizure initiation regions implicated in efficacy and avoiding those implicated in the effects on memory (Nobler et al. 1994; Sackeim et al. 2000a).

MST is a form of transcranial magnetic stimulation (TMS). The most common clinical and research use of TMS involves the repeated administration of trains of magnetic pulses to discrete brain regions without producing a seizure (George et al. 1999). Through induction of repeated pulses of current flow in underlying tissue, TMS can increase or decrease the excitability of underlying brain regions and thereby modulate activity in connected circuits (Paus et al. 1998). Numerous imaging studies and other work have demonstrated anatomical specificity in the neural regions dysregulated in major forms of psychopathology, especially major depression (Drevets 2000). Perhaps more consequential for the development of focal brain stimulation, there appears to be considerable consistency in the brain networks where changes in functional activity (i.e., excitation and inhibition) are associated with therapeutic response to antidepressant treatments (Drevets et al. 2002; Mayberg 2003; Nobler et al. 1994, 2001). Thus it is plausible that a nonconvulsive intervention that focally modulates functional brain activity can have therapeutic properties (Sackeim 2000).

Deep brain stimulation (DBS) builds on the notion that focal modulation of brain activity can be used therapeutically. DBS is the most focal and controlled of the brain stimulation techniques. In DBS, electrodes are implanted in a targeted nucleus and extended electrical stimulation is delivered directly to the tissue. In the case of movement disorders, the treatment can have an immediate effect on behavior. This therapeutic effect occurs because DBS takes a brain region "offline" and consequently, through patterns of connectivity, inhibits or disinhibits distal regions (Vesper et al. 2002; Vitek 2002).

In short, the fundamental concept underlying development of new brain stimulation techniques in psychiatry—MST, TMS, and DBS—is anatomical specificity in the neural regions that serve therapeutic response. In a simple world, the neural systems dysregulated in the major forms of psychopathology and those altered with successful treatment would be overlapping, if not identical. Thus, antidepressant treatments would reverse the abnormalities in functional brain activity that are characteristic of major depression. However, there is no necessary link between the biological disturbances that accompany or produce an illness and the biological alterations that modify expression of the illness and result in symptomatic improvement. In the case of major depression, there is consistent evidence that symptomatic improvement with classic treatments such as ECT and pharmacotherapy is accompanied by changes in brain physiology, but these changes do not involve reversal of baseline deficits (Nobler et al. 1994, 2000).

DBS for Parkinson's disease is a clear example of dissociation between the anatomy of illness and the anatomy of therapeutics. The circuitry involved in the etiology of Parkinson's disease is well characterized (DeLong et al. 1984), the ultimate cause being loss of dopamine-producing cells in the substantia nigra. As shown in Figure 5–1A, under normal circumstances, output of the substantia nigra pars compacta results in stimulation of dopamine D_1 and D_2 receptors in the putamen, which also receives excitatory input from the cortex. Outflow from the putamen affects the balance of excitation and inhibition in the external segment of the globus pallidus, subthalamic nucleus, internal segment of the globus pallidus, and the substantia nigra pars reticulata. The major efferent fibers from the basal ganglia, derived from the internal segment of the globus pallidus and substantia nigra pars reticulata, project to parts of the ventral anterior and ventral lateral thalamic nuclei. Excitatory output from ventral anterior/ventral lateral nuclei modulates activity in prefrontal and premotor cortices. This projection is the major outflow of the basal ganglia. Through this impact on cortical activity, the basal ganglia influence descending motor systems by way of cortical efferents to the brainstem (corticobulbar) and spinal cord (corticospinal). As Figure 5–1A shows, in normal functioning, inhibitory output from the internal segment of the globus pallidus and substantia nigra pars reticulata modulates excitatory input from the ventral anterior and ventral lateral nuclei to the cortex.

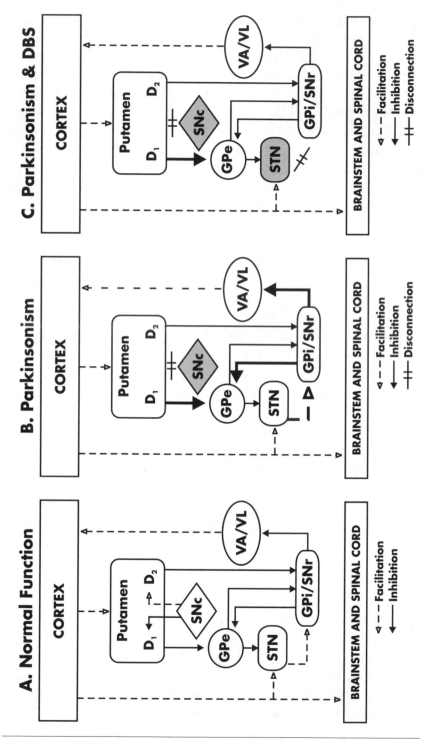

Figure 5–1. Key circuitry in the motor system, disruption by Parkinson's disease, and the effects of deep brain stimulation (DBS) delivered to the subthalamic nucleus (STN).

(A) depicts the excitatory and inhibitory influences under normal conditions. (B) shows the effects of Parkinson's disease and the loss of dopaminergic input from the substantia nigra pars compacta (SNc) to the putamen. This loss results ultimately in increased inhibitory output from the internal segment of the globus pallidus (GPi) and the substantia nigra pars reticulata (SNr) to the ventral anterior (VA) and ventral lateral (VL) thalamic nuclei. In turn, the facilitatory effect of VA and VL on the cortex is reduced. (C) The effects of DBS in Parkinson's disease when treatment is delivered to the STN are depicted. Output from VA and VL to the cortex is normalized. In (B) and (C) an increase in the thickness of lines indicates increased facilitation or inhibition. D_1, D_2 = dopamine receptors in the putamen; GPe = external segment of the globus pallidus.

Source. Models adapted from Delong et al. 1984.

In Parkinson's disease (Figure 5–1B), loss of dopaminergic transmission from the substantia nigra pars compacta to the putamen increases inhibitory outflow to the external segment of the globus pallidus. Through the described pattern of connectivity, excitatory input to the internal segment of the globus pallidus and substantia nigra pars reticulata increases, producing increased inhibition of ventral anterior/ventral lateral nuclei. The results are decreased excitatory input to the cortex and the classic signs of parkinsonism (resting tremor, bradykinesia, and rigidity).

The most well-studied use of DBS in Parkinson's disease involves stimulation of the subthalamic nucleus (Figure 5–1C), although therapeutic effects also have been obtained with chronic DBS in the globus pallidus. The subthalamic nucleus is not the site of the primary abnormality (Figure 5–1) in this degenerative disease and is only secondarily dysregulated. Rather, DBS, involving rapid and intense stimulation at approximately 185 Hz, is akin to taking the subthalamic nucleus offline or producing a subthalamic nuclear lesion (Haslinger et al. 2003). This removal of subthalamic nucleus outflow results in a chain of events reflecting decreased excitatory input to the internal segment of the globus pallidus and substantia nigra pars reticulata, increased excitation of ventral anterior and ventral lateral nuclei, and, consequently, an increase in excitatory signaling to the cortex.

The concept that brain interventions with therapeutic effects need not modify, let alone reverse, baseline abnormalities may apply more broadly than to the newer brain stimulation techniques alone. For example, to my knowledge, no one has experienced major depression because he or she has been "seizure deficient," yet ECT is our most effective short-term antidepressant, and the generalized seizure is a necessary but not sufficient condition for efficacy (Sackeim et al. 2000b).

That the neuroanatomical or neurophysiological bases of psychiatric disorders may be dissociated from processes involved in therapeutic effects does not weaken the rationale for the new brain stimulation techniques. The raison d'être for MST, TMS, and DBS is to intervene in a more spatially focal manner than had been previously possible, so as to modulate neurochemistry and functional activity in specific neural circuits and produce symptomatic relief (Sackeim 1994). Almost all psychotherapies have offered notions about the genesis of psychopathology based on observations of the mechanisms of therapeutic change. Similarly, major biological theories of pathoetiology, such as the dopamine hypothesis of schizophrenia and the catecholamine hypothesis of mood disorders, derived from beliefs about the mechanisms of therapeutic effects. These leaps often were not justified. Indeed, this type of unitary perspective was seemingly contradicted by the widespread view that the major psychiatric disorders are heterogeneous with regard to pathophysiological and etiological processes yet often show consistent response to biological interventions. When interventions affect a final common pathway, it is possible that diverse conditions with distinct developmental histories will show consistent improvement.

The disjunction between mechanisms of illness and therapeutics is particularly apparent in the case of VNS. It is not believed that epilepsy or major depression or almost any other possible indication for VNS results from an abnormality of the vagus nerve or insufficient stimulation of this nerve. Rather, VNS is used as a vehicle for modulating neurochemistry and brain activity in distributed regions.

VNS involves a surgical procedure in which a pulse generator or stimulator, akin to a cardiac pacemaker, is implanted under the skin of the anterior thorax and an electrode pair is attached to the vagus nerve (tenth cranial nerve) in the neck. Chronic stimulation is given, the most common paradigm involving 30 seconds of "on" time followed by 5 minutes of rest. Treatment continues 24 hours per day for months and years. Most of us had been taught that the vagus nerve plays a critical role in parasympathetic outflow from the brain, regulating peripheral function, especially in the heart and stomach. Why then consider VNS as a form of brain stimulation, as opposed, for instance, to an indirect method of regulating cardiac function? The other brain stimulation techniques, including ECT, are not wedded to particular circuitry. Depending on need, sites of stimulation can be altered with ECT, MST, TMS, and DBS, simply with changes in the positioning of electrodes (ECT, DBS) or the positioning or geometry of magnetic coils. Even with ECT, the least focal of these techniques, the efficacy and cognitive side effects of the treatment are strongly determined by the anatomical positioning of stimulating electrodes (e.g., unilateral versus bilateral ECT) and the extent to which electrical dosage exceeds seizure threshold (Sackeim et al. 1993, 2000b). In contrast, VNS is restricted to stimulating a single cranial nerve. Why was the vagus nerve selected and what are the consequences of VNS?

Brief History

For nearly a century, scientists have tested the possibility that the vagus nerve can serve as a portal for modulation of brain activity. This tack was taken because approximately 80% of fibers in the vagus nerve are afferent to higher brain centers, providing the central nervous system with visceral feedback from the head, neck, thorax, and abdomen. In early work, investigators tried to identify the extensive projections of the vagus nerve along its sensory afferent connections in the nucleus tractus solitarius (NTS) and from there to diverse brain regions (Figure 5–2). Documenting the changes in distal brain electrical activity that resulted from VNS was the prototypic paradigm for identifying this circuitry (Bailey and Bremer 1938; Dell and Olson 1951; MacLean 1990). Bailey and Bremer (1938) found that VNS in cats elicited synchronized activity in frontal orbital cortex. MacLean and Pribram, pioneers in neuroscience for other reasons, in 1949 recorded electroencephalographic activity from the cortical surface of anesthetized monkeys and found inconsistent slow waves generated from the lateral frontal cortex with VNS (MacLean 1990). Ruling out indirect brain changes due to efferent stimulation to the periphery, Dell and Olson (1951) reported that VNS produced electroencephalographic slow waves in the anterior rhinal sulcus and amygdala in awake cats with high cervical spinal section.

The key development for therapeutic application of VNS stemmed from preclinical research by Zabara (1985a, 1985b). The earlier findings indicated that VNS produced desynchronization of brain electrical activity with induction of slow waves. Slow, rhythmic electroencephalographic activity usually is interpreted

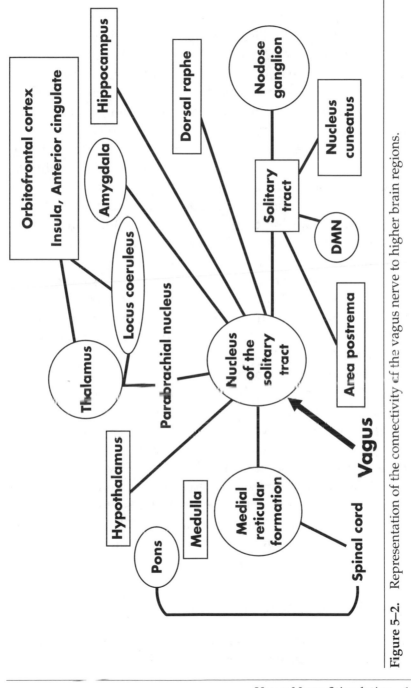

Figure 5–2. Representation of the connectivity of the vagus nerve to higher brain regions.

as indicating increased inhibitory tone (Sackeim et al. 1996). Given these findings and the projections of the vagus nerve to the NTS and then to diverse cortical and subcortical brain regions, Zabara determined whether VNS exerted anticonvulsant effects. Using experimental seizures in dogs, he found that VNS aborted ongoing ictal activity (Zabara 1992). Zabara hypothesized that VNS could serve two roles: 1) short-term intervention that would prevent (acute prophylactic effect) or stop (acute abortive effect) seizures owing to the immediate physiological impact of stimulation and 2) possible long-term treatment, in which tonic inhibition would increase with time owing to persistent effects of VNS (chronic progressive prophylactic effect) (Henry 2002). In the experimental model, Zabara found that the period of the anticonvulsant effect outlasted the period of short-term stimulation, theoretically supporting the possibility that intervention might be developed that had clinically significant long-term benefit.

In 1988, Penry treated the first patient with VNS as part of a pilot study with patients who had treatment-resistant epilepsy (partial seizure) and were not surgical candidates (Penry and Dean 1990). This treatment was soon followed by others (Rutecki 1990). Based primarily on the results of two pivotal, randomized, multisite trials (Ben-Menachem et al. 1994; George et al. 1994; Handforth et al. 1998; Ramsay et al. 1994; Vagus Nerve Stimulation Study Group 1995), the VNS Therapy System (formerly known as the NeuroCybernetic Prosthesis and developed by Cyberonics, Houston, TX) was approved in 1997 by the U.S. Food and Drug Administration (FDA) and labeled as adjunctive treatment for adults and adolescents older than 12 years with treatment-resistant partial-onset seizures. The system first became commercially available in Europe in 1994, also for treatment of this condition. Worldwide, approximately 20,000 people have undergone implantation of a vagus nerve stimulator for treatment of epilepsy.

Vagus Nerve Anatomy

The vagus nerve, or cranial nerve X, is mixed and consists of approximately 80% sensory fibers that are afferent to the brain, delivering information from the head, neck, thorax, and abdomen (George et al. 2000b). The sensory afferent cell bodies of the vagus nerve are in the nodose ganglion and relay information to the NTS (see Figure 5–2). The NTS has multiple and widespread projections to brainstem, limbic, and cortical areas. The projections involve three main pathways: 1) an autonomic feedback loop; 2) direct projections to the reticular formation in the medulla; and 3) ascending projections to the higher centers, largely through intermediaries in the parabrachial nucleus and the locus coeruleus. The parabrachial nucleus is adjacent to the locus coeruleus (the primary norepinephrine-containing area of the brain). Lesioning the locus coeruleus in rats appears to block the anticonvulsant effects of VNS, a finding that suggests stimulation of the locus coeruleus and increased noradrenergic transmission contribute to the antiepileptic properties of VNS (Krahl et al. 1998).

The parabrachial nucleus/locus coeruleus complex projects directly to various forebrain structures, specifically the hypothalamus, and several thalamic regions that modulate functional activity in the insula, orbitofrontal, and prefrontal cortex. The parabrachial nucleus/locus coeruleus complex is connected with the amygdala and the bed nucleus of the stria terminalis, brain regions long implicated in mood regulation, particularly states of fear and anxiety.

A series of preclinical studies with animals and brain imaging studies in patients has illustrated the functional consequences of this connectivity. For example, the oncogene c-*fos* is a marker of cellular stimulation or activity. VNS in rats enhances expression of this early gene in the amygdala, cingulate gyrus, locus coeruleus, and hypothalamus (Gieroba and Blessing 1994; Naritoku et al. 1995; Yousfi-Malki and Puizillout 1994) in a manner compatible with the anatomical projections. In imaging studies of the acute effects of VNS, patients with epilepsy underwent positron emission tomography (Henry 2000; Henry et al. 1998, 1999; Ko et al. 1996) and single-photon emission computed tomography (Ring et al. 2000; Van Laere et al. 2000, 2002; Vonck et al. 2000), and patients with major depression or epilepsy underwent functional magnetic resonance imaging (Bohning et al.

2001; George et al. 2003; Narayanan et al. 2002). The results demonstrated regional modulation of functional brain activity by VNS, large effects occurring in widely distributed regions. However, the findings have been complex in that the parameters of stimulation, especially overall intensity or charge, may modulate acute effects, and acute changes may differ in patients with epilepsy who do have a therapeutic response in terms of improved seizure frequency (Henry et al. 1999).

That VNS modulates the function of a fairly well-established set of brain regions is important in understanding its neurochemical effects and possible mechanisms in the treatment of seizure disorders and major depression. The NTS receives primary projections from the vagus nerve and projects on to widespread regions. Walker and colleagues (1999) found that injecting either γ-aminobutyric acid (GABA) agonists or glutamate antagonists into the NTS blocked seizures. This finding indirectly raised the possibility that VNS alters transmission in these inhibitory or excitatory systems. Krahl et al. (1998) found that inactivation of the locus coeruleus abolished the antiseizure effects of VNS. This finding suggested norepinephrine released with stimulation of this region contributed to anticonvulsant properties. Enhancement of noradrenergic transmission would also be compatible with antidepressant effects. Through projections from the NTS, VNS also results in stimulation of the dorsal raphe nucleus. In patients with epilepsy who underwent lumbar puncture studies, Ben-Menachem et al. (1995) found an increase in cerebral spinal fluid level of 5-hydroxyindoleacetic acid, the major metabolite of serotonin. If this change reflected increased serotonergic transmission, this finding was compatible with VNS exertion of antidepressant effects.

VNS is distinct from MST, TMS, and DBS, the other new brain stimulation techniques being explored as treatments of psychiatric disorders, in that VNS, by definition, is confined to stimulating one pathway, the vagus nerve. Nonetheless, it is evident that there are widespread anatomical projections from this cranial nerve and its major way station to the brain, the NTS. In line with this anatomy, imaging studies have shown that short-term VNS exerts marked effects on multiple brain regions, cortical and subcortical, and that these effects are dosage dependent. In particular, effects in the thalamus have been especially robust (Henry et al. 1999; Narayanan et al. 2002). It is well established that specific thalamic nuclei modulate electrical activity in widespread cortical regions (Dossi et al. 1992; Steriade 1994). Thus it is not surprising that early researchers found VNS resulted in synchronized slow-wave activity in prefrontal cortex (Bailey and Bremer 1938; MacLean 1990; MacLean and Pribram 1949).

Administration of Vagus Nerve Stimulation

VNS involves a surgical procedure that can be performed on an inpatient or outpatient basis. A neurosurgeon or vascular surgeon, with anesthesiologist support, usually conducts the procedure. Because the stimulator is tested during the surgical procedure (leads test), the physician who has prescribed and will be administering and monitoring VNS may also attend. This physician usually is a neurologist or psychiatrist.

The procedure involves placing a subcutaneous pulse generator in the chest wall and electrodes over the left vagus nerve. The NCP Pulse Generator can be externally programmed with respect to the key features of ultrabrief pulse stimulation (current amplitude, pulse width, pulse frequency, intertrain interval). Since the introduction of VNS as a therapeutic tool, pulse generators, which are much like cardiac pacemakers, have become smaller, and they have a long battery life. The generators, made of titanium, house a single battery that has an expected life of more than 7 years (depending on usage) before another surgical procedure is necessary for replacement.

The generator is implanted subcutaneously over the left chest wall, and another incision is made over the left vagus nerve in the neck. Bipolar helical electrodes are wrapped around the left vagus nerve near the carotid artery. To complete the circuit, leads connecting the generator and electrodes are tunneled under the skin between the incisions. The procedure typically takes 1.5 to 2 hours.

The implanted device is controlled by a magnetic wand attached to a portable computer. This system tests the integrity of the stimulation and sets the stimulus output parameters. The computer-controlled magnetic wand can interrogate the generator and store on the computer complete information about each pulse delivered since last interrogation. Future treatment delivery can be noninvasively programmed, and the parameters of the stimulation delivered can be documented precisely. After implantation, it is customary in both clinical practice and research to wait a short period (e.g., 1–2 weeks) before starting active stimulation.

Given that VNS involves an implanted device, there is no issue of compliance. Unless electrodes detach from the generator or the vagus nerve, delivered stimulation corresponds to received stimulation. Across medicine, lack of adherence to treatment regimens (noncompliance) is frequent and is often a key factor in reducing therapeutic effectiveness. Moreover, comorbid depression has been identified across a variety of primary disorders as pivotal in increasing lack of adherence with treatment (DiMatteo et al. 2000). That VNS almost guarantees full adherence is a distinct advantage, especially in the care of patients with severe depression or those who otherwise would undergo complex pharmacological regimens.

The prescribed VNS stimulus schedule need not always correspond to the stimulation parameters administered. This is one reason it is wise to retrieve and inspect information about the delivered stimulation. Each patient is given a small magnet that when placed on the skin over the generator suspends VNS. In other words, patients can turn off stimulation at any time for reasons of safety and convenience. For example, hoarseness and coughing are common side effects. VNS also can change the pitch of the voice during the periods of stimulus delivery. Therefore some patients prefer to turn off stimulation during public engagements. Likewise, patients with shortness of breath as a side effect may prefer to block stimulation during heavy exercise.

In the other direction, patients can use the magnet to deliver extra stimulation on demand. Swiping the magnet across the generator results in delivery of an additional pulse train. Patients with seizure disorders sometimes can tell that a seizure is imminent on the basis of prodromal signs and symptoms (i.e., aura).

The effect of this feature on seizure frequency and expression has not been systematically investigated, although some patients claim that delivering extra stimulation can block seizures or reduce their intensity. Regardless of the impact of seizures, one would expect this feature to have psychological effects. Pharmacotherapy-resistant seizure disorders can be considered prototypic examples of the conditions that foster learned helplessness because seizure occurrence often is unpredictable and uncontrollable. However, the on-demand feature has been disabled in all the work to date on VNS in the treatment of major depression. Because major depression does not involve a punctate event that hypothetically can be blocked, the capacity to self-administer additional rounds of stimulation seems unjustified. Furthermore, falsely empowering patients in this way can confound assessment of the effects of VNS on major depression.

The prototypic VNS protocol in neurological and psychiatric disorders involves delivering a pulse train for 30 seconds at full amplitude followed by a 5-minute rest period, the on and off periods repeated continuously 24 hours a day. As Figure 5–3 shows, the period of full stimulation (on time) is preceded by a 2-second ramp up of the output current and followed by a 2-second ramp down. The physician prescribing VNS has the option of varying numerous parameters, the most critical of which are pulse amplitude or current, pulse frequency (reciprocal of interpulse interval), pulse width, train duration (on time), and intertrain interval (off time).

When patients first receive active VNS, after recovery from the surgical procedure, they start with a period of pulse amplitude titration. The current administered during each pulse is progressively increased during the first few visits to a level comfortable for the patient. Although voice alteration may be prominent during stimulation (on time), dyspnea, interference with swallowing, or painful sensations indicate excessive current. Because tolerance develops for many VNS side effects, adjustments to current intensity may be made over the first several weeks of treatment.

VNS has numerous electrical and timing parameters and almost limitless permutations. Consequently, determining for clin-

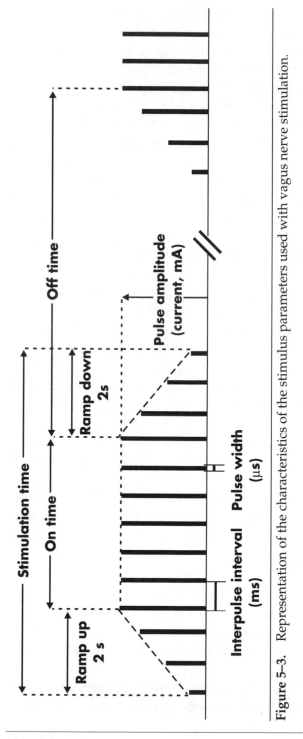

Figure 5–3. Representation of the characteristics of the stimulus parameters used with vagus nerve stimulation.

ical use which sets of parameters yield the greatest benefit/risk ratios is difficult, and no large-scale studies with systematically varying single parameters have been conducted for any disorder. Rather, in randomized, multicenter trials of treatment of epilepsy, patients were assigned to either low- or high-stimulation conditions, which differed in pulse frequency, pulse width, and duty cycle. In the first randomized trial (E03), a robust difference at the immediate study end point favored more intensive stimulation for beneficial effects on seizure control (Vagus Nerve Stimulation Study Group 1995). Although there were indications of a similar effect in the second randomized trial (E05), the differences between the conditions were not robust (Handforth et al. 1998). Thus although there is evidence that more intensive stimulation may result in better seizure control, the role of individual parameters, the shape of the dose/response function, and many other key issues require study.

What has been learned from the work in epilepsy and major depression derives mainly from naturalistic observation, a search for associations between variation in stimulus parameters and therapeutic or adverse effects. No aspect of stimulus delivery has been found related to the anticonvulsant or antidepressant properties of VNS (Amar et al. 1999; Morris and Mueller 1999; Sackeim et al. 2001c). In general, excessive stimulus intensity, especially with respect to pulse amplitude (current) but also reflected in pulse width or frequency, is thought to be key to the severity of side effects (Ben-Menachem 2001; Binnie 2000; Charous et al. 2001). In the two randomized trials in epilepsy, voice alteration was more frequent among patients randomized to high than to low intensity, with a similar effect for dyspnea in E05 (Handforth et al. 1998; Ramsay et al. 1994). However, other side effects did not show this difference.

Complicating the issue is that pulse amplitude is titrated to a clinically relevant, but immeasurable, end point: patient's report that the level of stimulation is as high as is comfortably tolerable. Wide individual differences have been observed in the pulse amplitudes reached with this approach. In the first study in major depression (D01), pulse amplitude during the short-term trial period varied across the 59 evaluable patients from

0.25 to 3.0 milliamperes (Sackeim et al. 2001c), a 12-fold range. Undoubtedly, some of this variability is due to anatomical factors, reflecting individual differences in vagus nerve anatomy and the positioning and fit of the electrodes (Woodbury and Woodbury 1990, 1991). However, individuals vary considerably in the extent to which they find side effects tolerable. It was noteworthy that the average level of stimulation in this trial was higher than that in the controlled studies in epilepsy. The investigators believed that a number of depressed patients accepted uncomfortable levels of stimulation because of their conviction that more intense stimulation would have greater efficacy.

If VNS is effective at all in neuropsychiatric disorders, there must be dose/response relationships between aspects of stimulus intensity and behavioral effects. Unlike VNS, ECT involves direct stimulation to broad central nervous system areas and produces a seizure, fundamentally altering the physiological state of the brain. Nonetheless, it is well established that the efficacy of ECT in major depression is highly contingent on the current paths in the brain and the current density within those paths (McCall et al. 2000; Sackeim et al. 1993, 2000b). VNS, because of its restriction to a single nerve bundle for direct stimulation, and without the complication of a seizure, should provide greater opportunity for parameterization. For example, in examining the anticonvulsant properties of VNS, Woodbury and Woodbury (1990) reported that maximal stimulation of vagal C fibers at frequencies greater than 4 Hz prevented or reduced chemically and electrically induced seizures in young male rats. The anticonvulsant effects were related to the fraction of vagal C fibers stimulated. Optimal parameters included pulse frequency between 10 and 20 Hz and a pulse amplitude of 0.2–0.5 milliamperes per square millimeter of the nerve cross section. Results of experiments with animals suggested that the effects of VNS in modifying seizure expression depend on dosage parameters in a specific fiber group. Were telemetric recording possible during and after VNS trains, indices of the immediate physiological effects of stimulation could be obtained and used as a method of dosage adjustment.

Vagus Nerve Stimulation in Treatment-Resistant Epilepsy

Despite the widespread availability of second and third generation antiepileptic drugs (AEDs), many patients with partial-onset
seizures do not benefit fully or have side effects that limit the utility of pharmacotherapy. Several nonpharmacological treatments,
such as tissue resection and electrical stimulation of the thalamus
or cerebellum, have been explored as adjuncts or alternatives to
pharmacotherapy. Although study of such treatments has taken
on new life with investigations of the use of DBS in epilepsy, until
recently only neurosurgery was widely considered safe and effective in the care of adults with resistant partial-onset seizure
disorders. However, the number of patients who undergo surgical resection is a small fraction of those with poor or inadequate
seizure control. Many resistant patients are not candidates for resection owing to the presence of multiple foci, the location of foci,
and concern about the consequences and cost of surgery.

The first two research trials of VNS in epilepsy (E01, E02)
were conducted with open-label, naturalistic, longitudinal de-
signs and involved treatment of 15 patients with medication-
resistant partial-onset seizures (Penry and Dean 1990). Approval
of the treatment by the FDA was primarily based on results of
two pivotal trials (E03, E05) in which 313 patients with resistant
partial-onset seizures received stimulation after being randomized to low- or high-intensity conditions (Handforth et al. 1998;
Vagus Nerve Stimulation Study Group 1995). In addition, a
larger open-label, longitudinal study (E04) was conducted with
patients who had a variety of seizures disorders; E04 also included children (Labar et al. 1999, 2000).

Studies E03 and E05 provided the key data on the efficacy of
VNS in patients with treatment-resistant, partial-onset seizure
disorder. Both were multicenter studies that used a randomized,
masked, active control design. Patients were observed over a 12–
16-week baseline period, during which changes in AED dosage
were kept to a minimum and the seizure rate determined. Patients who met inclusion criteria at the end of the baseline period
underwent implantation of the device and, after a 2-week recov-

ery interval, were randomly assigned to either a low- or a high-stimulation condition. The low-stimulation intervention, which was hypothesized to be less effective, delivered 1-Hz stimulation with a 130-microsecond pulse width for 30 seconds on time and 90–180 minutes off time. In contrast, the high-stimulation condition delivered 30-Hz pulse frequency with 500-microsecond pulse width for 30 seconds on time and 5 minutes off time. A methodological limitation, possibly compromising the masking, was inequality in how pulse amplitude (current) was determined for the low- and high-stimulation groups. During the first 2 weeks after randomization, the high-stimulation patients had amplitude adjusted to the highest level tolerated. In the low-stimulation group, titration was only to the level that patients could perceive. Immediate outcome was assessed throughout the subsequent 12 weeks of short-term treatment.

In both E03 and E05, patients on average had a more than 20-year history of seizure disorder. On average they were taking slightly more than two AEDs daily, having tried and discontinued more than five other AEDs in the past. Pharmacotherapy was kept constant throughout the short-term trial period, and VNS was tested as adjunctive therapy, which is now the routine method in evaluation of new AEDs. The primary outcome measure in these trials was mean percentage reduction in seizure frequency. At the end of the short-term treatment period, the high-stimulation group in E03 averaged a 24.5% reduction in seizure frequency compared with 6.1% for the low-stimulation condition. For E05 the comparable rates of reduction were 28% and 15%. Immediate response was defined as at least a 50% reduction in symptom scores. The response rates in E03 were 31% and 13% for the high- and low-stimulation groups, respectively. Although this comparison was not significant in E05, the proportion of patients with at least 75% reduction in seizures was greater in the high- than the low-stimulation group (11% versus 2%).

These findings of greater reduction in seizure frequency in high- than in low-stimulation conditions supported the notion that VNS exerts anticonvulsant effects. Use of an active comparison (low-stimulation condition) made this claim more credible than would comparison with treatment as usual (AEDs alone) or a sham intervention that did not involve stimulation of the vagus nerve. Nonetheless, in these studies very few patients became seizure free. Even the response rates at the end of the short-term trial, defined as 50% reduction in seizure frequency, were modest in the high-stimulation groups (E03, 31%; E05, 23%). Therefore it could be questioned whether an intervention that required surgery and device implantation should be widely considered when the short-term benefits appeared to be so limited.

Long-Term Therapeutic Effects in Epilepsy

Each of the five studies (E01–E05) that were the original examinations of the short-term effects of VNS in patients with medication-resistant epilepsy contained a longitudinal follow-up component. During follow-up study, concomitant treatment was not controlled. With notable consistency, the findings within and across these studies suggested that seizure frequency continues to decrease as time from implantation increases, although such improvement may level off between 1 and 2 years into the follow-up period. Figure 5–4 presents the response rates over time (≥50% reduction in seizure frequency relative to pre-VNS baseline) totaled across 440 participants in five studies (Morris and Mueller 1999). This rate increased from 23% 3 months after implantation to 43% at both 2 and 3-year follow-up evaluations, essentially doubling the number of patients who had a substantial degree of reduction of seizure frequency.

In long-term follow-up studies, other aspects of treatment were uncontrolled, particularly type and dosage of AEDs. Changes in AED treatment regimens were common, and it is hazardous to conclude that continued improvement during the follow-up period reflected progressive or late effects of VNS. On the other hand, many clinicians are convinced that long-term improvement in seizure control and other dimensions, such as quality of life, is attributable to VNS. This view is derived from the experience that some patients had relapses when VNS was stopped or reduced in intensity and from the uniform lack of improvement during a long history of treatment with various AED combinations (Amar et al. 1999). Regardless, there is little prece-

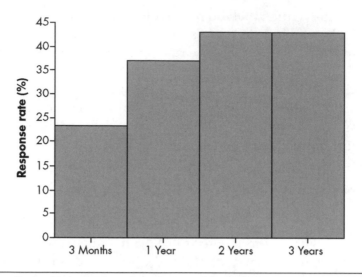

Figure 5–4. Percentage of patients with treatment-resistant epilepsy meeting response criteria 3 months and 1, 2, and 3 years after starting vagus nerve stimulation.

Source. Data from Morris and Mueller 1999.

dent for a treatment in neuropsychiatry that has the inverse of a tolerance effect, that is, greater long-term than short-term efficacy. In the treatment of major depression, we are familiar with the "poop out" that can occur with use of selective serotonin reuptake inhibitors. Our most powerful antidepressant treatment, ECT, is remarkable in the short term but carries a high risk of relapse (Sackeim et al. 2001a). Thus the possibility of sustained, long-term improvement would certainly justify consideration of VNS, as long as side effects are acceptable. The suggestion of sustained long-term benefit in epilepsy was one of the factors that prompted study of VNS for treatment-resistant major depression, often a chronic, unremitting disorder. However, caution is especially needed when uncontrolled, open studies yield findings that are counterintuitive and clinically exciting. No matter what our convictions, only controlled research can establish whether VNS has the unusual property of being more effective years after the start of treatment than in the first several months. The time scale at issue, in which benefit is maximal 1 to 2 years after the start of treatment, does not conform to our understanding of the time course of the physiological and neuroanatomical changes that may mediate these behavioral effects. In other words, if VNS exerts these very late beneficial effects, we are at a loss to explain how this occurs.

The pivotal E03 and E05 studies focused on adults with medication-resistant partial-onset seizures. Other work examined the efficacy of VNS in the treatment of epileptic children 12 years of age and younger and in persons with seizure disorders other than partial onset. The evidence to date suggests that children with seizure disorders are similar to adults in extent and quality of improvement (Labar 2000; Murphy 1999; Nagarajan et al. 2002). Likewise, results of naturalistic studies have suggested that VNS has beneficial effects on seizure disorders other than those with partial onset, including generalized epilepsy characterized by mixed generalized seizures (Labar et al. 1999).

Results of two controlled trials suggested that VNS has stronger antiepileptic properties when administered at high relative to low stimulus intensity. However, the magnitude of this difference in immediate outcome was relatively modest in at least one of the two trials, and overall rates of response indicated that most of the patients had limited or no benefit after 12 weeks of treatment. In contrast, results of longitudinal, naturalistic follow-up studies revealed a substantial increase in response rate 1–2 years after initial implantation. In line with these data, the rate of discontinuation of VNS (i.e., explantation or surgical removal of the VNS stimulator) 1 and 2 years after implantation was remarkably low in these studies. This finding suggested that patients perceived sufficient benefit to justify continuing the intervention (Morris and Mueller 1999). Nonetheless, use of VNS in epilepsy varies considerably across institutions and practitioners, and its value has been hotly debated in neurology (Ben-Menachem 1998; McLachlan 1998). Some centers that rarely perform the procedure emphasize the small effect sizes in randomized comparisons of acute effects and the absence of controlled data on long-term benefit. Other clinicians are convinced that some patients who have exhausted or nearly exhausted pharmacological options have improvement, often after a substantial delay.

Rationale for Use of Vagus Nerve Stimulation in Major Depression

There has been considerable interest in the use of VNS for treatment-resistant psychiatric disorders, especially major depression. The rationale for exploring potential antidepressant effects of VNS was detailed by George et al. 2000a and includes several of its properties already described. The foremost is that VNS has marked anticonvulsant effects, as found in both basic research and treatment trials in epilepsy. A variety of anticonvulsant medications (e.g., carbamazepine, lamotrigine, and valproate) are used as mood stabilizers, or in the case of lamotrigine, as an antidepressant. The most effective antidepressant treatment, ECT, exerts powerful anticonvulsant properties, which have been linked to its efficacy in major depression (Sackeim 1999; Sackeim et al. 1983). Although tricyclic antidepressants and lithium can produce iatrogenic seizures when dosage is excessive, within the therapeutic range for treatment of mood disorders, these medications exert anticonvulsant effects, as revealed in both basic research and trials in epilepsy (Fromm et al. 1972; Shukla et al. 1988).

Another key consideration was the contention that the therapeutic effects in epilepsy showed the reverse of a tolerance effect, increasing with time since implantation. This concern was of special importance because a surgical implantation procedure that commonly results in voice alteration and coughing as side effects would hardly be desirable if antidepressant effects were only transient. Many patients with treatment-resistant depression have short-lived symptomatic improvement when new medication or ECT regimens are introduced. In light of the experience in epilepsy, VNS had the potential of providing a sustained therapeutic effect.

Another clinical consideration was the informal observation early in the trials in epilepsy that many patients reported improvement in mood independent of changes in seizure frequency or intensity. A small study of mood changes in patients treated with VNS for seizure disorders provided empirical support for this view (Harden et al. 2000).

The neurobiological effects of VNS also stimulated interest in its potential as an antidepressant treatment. VNS stimulates the locus coeruleus and the dorsal raphe, enhancing transmission of norepinephrine and serotonin, respectively (Ben-Menachem et al. 1995). As indicated earlier, VNS also modulates glutamatergic and GABAergic transmission. These neurochemical effects are compatible with classic theorizing about antidepressant mechanisms. As an additional rationale, some experts have emphasized the brain imaging findings in epilepsy, which indicate that the immediate effects of VNS involve alteration of functional activity across widely distributed brain regions (Henry 2002; Henry et al. 1998). However, these changes have been examined principally in terms of the immediate effects of stimulation on brain activity, whereas the capacity of VNS to make sustained alterations in brain activity is the more concerning issue. In addition, some authorities have interpreted the epilepsy work as demonstrating VNS effects specifically on the limbic structures involved in mood regulation. This type of statement is misleading, partly because we do not fully understand the circuitry of mood disorders and partly because the acute effects of VNS on functional brain activity are widely distributed, only partially overlapping in topography with the changes that accrue with response to established antidepressant treatments.

Efficacy in Major Depression: Study D01

On the basis of the rationale presented in the preceding section, an open-label, multisite pilot study (referred to as D01) was conducted to examine the safety and efficacy of VNS in major depression (Rush et al. 2000; Sackeim et al. 2001c). The sites were Baylor University (principal investigator, L. B. Marangell), Medical University of South Carolina (principal investigator, M. S. George), New York State Psychiatric Institute (principal investigator, H. A. Sackeim), and the University of Texas at Southwestern (principal investigator, A. J. Rush). The patients in this trial met the DSM-IV criteria for nonpsychotic major depressive episode (American Psychiatric Association 1994), either unipolar or bipolar, but rapid-cycling was excluded. Inclusion criteria required that all patients have evidence of significant treatment resistance, having shown inadequate response to at least two antidepressant trials in the current episode as defined by the Antidepressant Treatment History Form (Sackeim 2001). In addition, patients had to meet the DSM-IV criteria for either recurrent or chronic major depressive episode.

The goal in the design of the study was to recruit patients who had not benefited sufficiently from robust antidepressant treatment trials and who, given this history, had few treatment options that had a reasonable likelihood of success. Reflecting this intent, at baseline the average duration of a current major depressive episode among the 60 patients who entered this trial was nearly 10 years (median, 6.6 years), a remarkable degree of chronicity for a mood disorder group. The average score on the 28-item Hamilton Rating Scale for Depression (Ham-D) was 36.8 (SD, 5.8), reflecting a degree of symptom severity greater than that seen in most inpatient studies of ECT. With respect to pharmacological and other somatic treatments, the sample averaged 16 distinct psychiatric interventions during the index episode, nine of which involved classic antidepressant trials. Approximately two-thirds of the patients had received ECT during the current episode, and on a lifetime basis, nearly all patients had been treated with this modality. With respect to formal Antidepressant Treatment History Form criteria for adequate antidepressant treatments, in the current episode 18 (30%) of the patients had not benefited from two adequate antidepressant trials, 4 (7%) had not benefited from three trials, 12 (20%) had not benefited from four trials, and 26 (43%) had not benefited from five or more trials.

Surgical implantation was performed after the medication stabilization period and baseline assessment. A single-masked 2-week recovery period immediately followed surgery. Patients were told that VNS may or may not be started after implantation, when, in fact, no stimulation was given. One of 60 patients improved sufficiently during the recovery period to no longer meet study inclusion criteria, and short-term efficacy was evaluated in the 59 patients who completed the study. During the first 2 weeks following the recovery period, the intensity of VNS was ramped up. During frequent visits at the site, pulse amplitude was progressively increased in a manner akin to the epilepsy trials, the goal being a tolerable stimulation dosage. Meeting this goal required multiple visits because tolerance develops rapidly to some of the adverse effects of VNS. After the adjustment phase, dosing remained fixed for the subsequent 10 weeks, during which there were frequent clinical evaluations. Patients in this study were eligible for long-term follow-up care involving safety and clinical evaluation at least quarterly and continuing indefinitely. Several years of follow-up evaluation have now accrued since the first patients with major depression underwent implantation.

Acute response was defined as 50% improvement in symptom score. Remission was defined as a score of 10 or less on the 28-item Ham-D. The response rates at short-term trial termination were 30.5% for the primary Ham-D measure, 34.0% for the Montgomery-Åsberg Depression Rating Scale, and 37.3% for the Clinical Global Impression–Improvement Scale (score of 1 or 2). The portion of the sample meeting remission criteria was 15.3%. During the acute phase, two patients became hypomanic. Nevertheless, given the degree of treatment resistance, chronicity, and symptom severity in the sample, it was deemed that clinical outcome at the end of the short-term treatment phase reflected clinically significant benefit (Sackeim et al. 2001c).

This impression was reinforced by the findings of the long-term naturalistic follow-up study (Marangell et al. 2002). A major confounding factor with the follow-up results was absence of control over changes in concomitant treatments. Thus it could not be determined whether the long-term effects observed were attributable to VNS or to institution of more effective pharmacological strategies or use of ECT. Nonetheless, examining the first 30 patients to enter the D01 study, Marangell et al. (2002) reported that the response rate increased to 46% when outcome at the end of the short-term trial was compared with that 9 months later (1 year after implantation). The remission rate increased to 29% over this time frame. The results are available for the total sample of subjects who completed the study—31% classified as responders after the acute phase and 45% so classified after 9 months of follow-up evaluation (unpublished data, September

2002). Thus, as for the findings in epilepsy, it appeared that clinical outcome improved with additional exposure to VNS. These changes in symptoms were accompanied, as expected, by improvements in function (Marangell et al. 2002). However, as in the epilepsy literature, alterations in treatment regimens other than VNS could not be ruled out as contributing to the improved status.

There were indications of site differences in the pilot D01 study. Clinical outcome was poorest at the New York State Psychiatric Institute/Columbia University site, where only 1 (8.3%) of 12 patients in D01 met response criteria at the end of the acute phase. This site was exceptional in having an independent board of expert pharmacologists review the treatment history of each patient to ensure reasonable options had been exhausted before study entry. Furthermore, the orientation was not simply to ensure that previous treatment was adequate in meeting the standard criteria for medication dose and duration. When treatment was tolerable, patients were encouraged to have especially potent trials before study entry.

Overall, the patients in New York tended to differ from those at the other sites in number of adequate treatment trials received in the current episode and lifetime, number of psychotropic medications (antidepressant or otherwise) received during the episode, and length of index episode. Relative to the other three sites, the patients at Columbia had a substantially greater history of treatment-resistant illness, and the current episode was of longer duration.

The site differences were consequential because they offered important clues regarding the clinical features that may be predictive of responsiveness to VNS in major depression. Sackeim et al. (2001b) examined a variety of clinical features and treatment variables as potential predictors of short-term clinical outcome of VNS. Most variables had no relationship to clinical outcome, including initial severity of symptoms and the intensity of VNS stimulation. The factor that showed the strongest and most consistent relationship to short-term outcome (later replicated in this sample for long-term outcome) was degree of treatment resistance. As shown in Figure 5–5, among the subgroup of patients

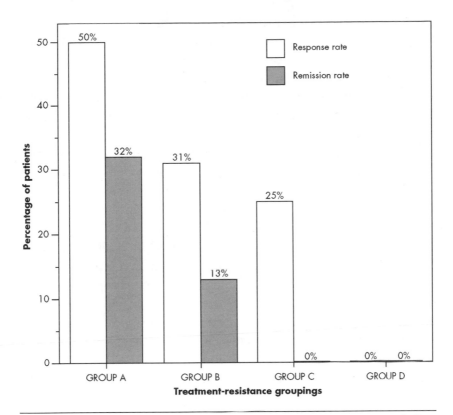

Figure 5–5. Response and remission rates for vagus nerve stimulation at the end of the short-term D01 trial period as a function of medication resistant grouping.

Group A had not responded to 2 or 3 adequate medication trials in the current episode, while Group D had not responded to 7 or more trials.

Source. Data from Sackeim et al. 2001c.

who had not responded to the largest number of adequate antidepressant trials during the index episode, no patient either responded or had remission (Sackeim et al. 2001c).

Contrary to the original hopes that VNS would be especially helpful for treatment of patients with the most resistant conditions, the findings of pilot study D01 suggested that the likelihood of benefit with VNS decreased linearly as treatment resistance increased. Furthermore, this relationship was seen in long-term follow-up evaluation of the D01 patients. Response status and remission status at 1 year were linked to degree of treatment resistance expressed during the index episode (Marangell et al. 2002). Nonetheless, it was evident that many patients who had not responded to two or more adequate trials benefited from VNS. The long-term findings were especially intriguing, suggesting that VNS might have persistent therapeutic effects—indeed, therapeutic effects that became enhanced with increasing long-term exposure.

The next exploration of VNS in major depression was a pivotal trial, conducted to obtain FDA approval to market the device as an intervention for treatment-resistant depression. VNS was well tolerated in this group, with side effects similar to those encountered by epilepsy patients. The most common side effect was voice alteration or hoarseness, occurring in 36 (60%) of 60 patients. The hoarseness was generally mild and related to the intensity of the output current. There were no adverse cognitive effects (Sackeim et al. 2001b).

Most interestingly, VNS as used in this open study was more effective in those depressed patients whose illness showed lower degrees of treatment resistance. For the group of 59 patients, a history of treatment resistance and intensity of concurrent antidepressant treatment during the short-term VNS trial were related to VNS outcome. For example, none of the 13 patients who had not responded adequately to more than seven research-defined adequate antidepressant trials in the current episode responded, but 18 (39%) of the remaining 46 patients did respond ($P=0.0057$) (Sackeim et al. 2001c).

Response rates at the end of the 10-week short-term phase appeared to largely continue and even improve over 9 months of long-term maintenance VNS treatment after exit from the short-term study (Marangell et al. 2002). Changes in psychotropic medications and in VNS stimulus parameters were allowed during this long-term follow-up period.

Efficacy in Major Depression: Studies D02 and D04

The next study, D02, also was sponsored by Cyberonics. After detailed presentation of the design and methods, the FDA agreed to consider it a pivotal study to be used as the key element in the Cyberonics application for postmarket approval. In other words, if the outcome of D02 was sufficiently positive in terms of both clinical benefit and safety, on the basis of the results of this study the FDA would consider approving VNS for routine use in the treatment of depression. Were the FDA to take this action, VNS would be the first nonpharmacological, somatic therapy for depression since ECT to receive FDA approval for routine use. At the time of this writing, the short-term treatment phase of D02 is complete. It has been at least 12 months since the last patient to enter the protocol completed the short-term phase. However, the D02 findings, although subject to considerable scrutiny by expert advisory committees and the press, are in the process of being submitted for publication. Accordingly, the following account of this study should be considered preliminary.

D02 had a randomized, double-masked, sham-controlled design for comparing the short-term efficacy and safety of active VNS (implantation plus continuous stimulation) and sham VNS (implantation without stimulation). The study design is illustrated in Figure 5–6. Inclusion and exclusion criteria were similar to those used in D01, with one major exception. On the basis of ratings on the Antidepressant Treatment History Form (Sackeim 2001), a cap was placed on the number of adequate medication trials patients received during the index episode and for which there was inadequate response. Patients who had not responded to seven or more adequate antidepressant trials were excluded from participation. This change in procedure from D01 was dictated by the findings regarding predictors of outcome and was intended to limit the number of participants who would be unlikely to benefit either immediately or in the long term. Another design innovation in D02 was use of a rater certification program and site- and time-masked ratings of videotapes of the key clinical interviews by experienced evaluators at Columbia University. With a new structured interview for the Ham-D, a specialized training and certification program, and ongoing feedback regarding the quality of interviews and scoring, near perfect reliability was obtained between the ratings conducted at the sites ($n > 20$) and the expert raters.

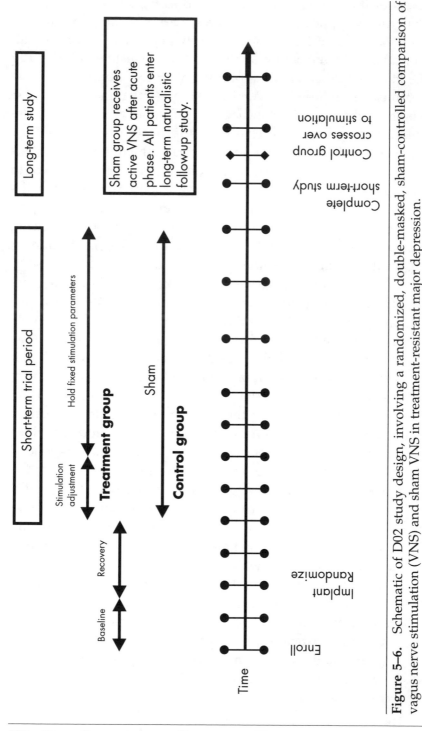

Figure 5–6. Schematic of D02 study design, involving a randomized, double-masked, sham-controlled comparison of vagus nerve stimulation (VNS) and sham VNS in treatment-resistant major depression.

According to the procedures for D01, all patients began a baseline period during which psychotropic medications were stabilized and study eligibility determined. For all patients, this period was followed by implantation and a recovery period during which patients were told they might or might not receive stimulation during the study. Patients who continued to meet inclusion/exclusion criteria after the 2-week recovery period were randomly assigned to active or sham VNS. At each site, only a VNS programmer knew the treatment group assignment (i.e., active versus sham). All patients were told they might or might not experience sensations during VNS delivery. An attempt was made to avoid contact among study participants, including scheduling non-overlapping time for study visits. The intention was to limit the extent to which participants shared experiences with VNS, and thus to preserve the integrity of the mask. The extent to which this barrier was implemented was unknown. When participants arrived for study visits, the stimulator was turned off, preserving the mask for study personnel other than the programmer. During the first 2 weeks after recovery, the active VNS group underwent adjustment of the stimulus output parameters, and the programmer mimicked this procedure in the sham patients. Except for adjustments due to side effects, stimulus parameters were kept constant during the remaining 10 weeks of the trial. After the short term phase, patients who received the sham intervention were offered the opportunity to receive active VNS. All patients then entered a long term naturalistic follow-up study.

The response rates, defined as a decrease of at least 50% in Ham-D score at the end of the short-term phase, were surprisingly low. Among patients receiving active VNS, the response rate was approximately 15%, whereas the rate was approximately 10% in the sham group. Across a variety of clinical outcome measures, with the exception of one self-report scale, there was no difference between the two intervention groups at the end of the randomized short-term phase. Relative to D01, patients receiving active VNS had considerably less improvement during and at the end of the acute phase.

The main intent of this study was to demonstrate that active treatment was superior to sham VNS in short-term antidepressant effects. This outcome did not occur, and the null hypothesis that active is not different from sham VNS in efficacy could not be rejected despite a substantial sample size. The reasons for this difference from D01, which had twice the response rate after open, immediate-phase treatment, were given scrutiny. One possible explanation is that stimulus output parameters were lower in D02 than in D01. The use of low-intensity stimulation may have resulted from an emphasis on preserving the mask and the belief that superior outcome is not achieved when parameters are more intense than those used in studies in which the patients have complex partial seizures. It is possible that a substantial number of patients received stimulation with an intensity below a threshold for obtaining response.

As in D01, there was an increase in response/remission rate when patients were examined 9 months after implantation and the start of active stimulation. Across the sample, the cross-sectional response rate was approximately 30%, combining the original active and sham VNS groups. Long-term clinical outcome was compared for D02 study participants and patients in a companion health-economics study (D04). In the D04 study, patients did not have a VNS stimulator implanted. Rather, they received routine clinical care (including medications and possibly ECT) but did not receive VNS. Patients in D04 could not participate in D02 because of logistical issues, study exclusion criteria, or closed enrollment in D02. In short, with the exception of implantation, D04 provided an estimate of clinical outcome effects with a similar sample receiving treatment as usual.

Across a variety of measures, there was a substantial difference in long-term clinical outcome favoring the D02 group, that is, patients who received VNS. In general, response and remission rates in the D04 sample were about one-half those in the D02 sample. At minimum, this finding indicated that standard interventions for patients with treatment-resistant major depression are typically ineffective and that symptomatic manifestation is prolonged. The superiority of VNS to treatment as usual has sparked great interest, and the claim of long-term benefit may be at the heart of a revised premarket approval effort. Clearly, any treatment that provides some measure of symptom relief and does so in a sustained manner is of great interest.

Although the recent findings that active VNS was superior to treatment as usual are important, several reservations about these findings should be kept in mind. First, there was no evidence that VNS was effective in short-term use in D02, the controlled study. It is highly unusual for an agent to exert antidepressant properties in the long but not the short term. In addition, the primary criterion for outcome, 50% reduction in symptoms, although common in industry-sponsored work, is weak. Especially among those with treatment-resistant conditions, who tend to have more severe pathologic findings, patients can have a condition that is highly symptomatic at trial conclusion but be classified as responders, owing to a high ceiling. Perhaps of greater concern is that the comparison of D02 and D04 was nonrandomized, and the representativeness of the D04 sample is unknown. Furthermore, it is unknown whether the two groups differed in key predictive variables such as extent of treatment resistance. Finally, the long-term response rate among D01 patients was just at the border of suggesting clinical utility.

Side Effects

In the studies with patients who had major depression, the types and rates of adverse events were similar to those observed in the studies with patients who had treatment-resistant epilepsy. There was no death in D01 during the short- or long-term followup phases. The most common side effects, as in epilepsy, included voice alteration, coughing, neck pain, and dyspnea (Marangell et al. 2002; Sackeim et al. 2001c). Tolerance to these side effects develops rapidly, and the frequency of adverse events is considerably lower during long-term treatment than after surgery or the start of short-term treatment. The mechanisms underlying tolerance are poorly understood, although side effects such as voice alteration probably reflect spread of current to the vocal cords. It is important to note that most patients find the side effects not bothersome. In D01, 59 of the 60 patients elected to continue VNS in the long-term follow-up study.

Several patients experienced hypomania or mania after introduction of VNS. Given that this is a well-known iatrogenic effect of some medications, it would be interesting to determine comparability in rates of this outcome for VNS and standard antidepressants. If , in fact, the hypomania was due to VNS, as opposed to natural cycling or medication alteration, that would be another indication that VNS acts as an antidepressant.

Because VNS has marked anticonvulsant effects and imaging findings established it has a widespread effect on functional brain activity, there has been the concern that, like ECT, VNS may result in cognitive compromise. There had been surprisingly little research on the neuropsychological sequelae of VNS in epilepsy, and the basic and clinical research findings in this area conflicted, suggesting decrements, no change, or improvement (Clark et al. 1998, 1999; Helmstaedter et al. 2001; Hoppe et al. 2001; Sjogren et al. 2002).

As part of the D01 study, my associates and I evaluated 27 of the first 30 patients with an extensive neuropsychological battery that was administered before active stimulation and at termination of the short-term treatment course (a 10-week interval) (Sackeim et al. 2001b). Thirteen neurocognitive tests were performed to sample the domains of motor speed, psychomotor function, language, attention, memory, and executive function. There was no evidence of deterioration in any neurocognitive measure over the short-term treatment phase. Relative to baseline, improvements in motor speed (finger tapping), psychomotor function (digit-symbol test), language (verbal fluency), and executive functions (logical reasoning, working memory, and response inhibition or impulsiveness) were found. As is often seen in depressed samples, for some measures, improved neurocognitive performance covaried with reduction in depressive symptoms, but VNS output current was not related to changes in cognitive performance. Thus the results of this study suggested that rather than being a safety concern, VNS for treatment-resistant depression may result in enhanced neurocognitive function, primarily among patients who have clinical improvement. However, controlled investigation is needed to rule out the contribution of practice effects.

The side effects of VNS are unusual compared with those of medications and ECT. For example, it may be initially disconcerting to patients and family members to hear the change in the patient's voice (increase in pitch) when stimulation is delivered. Nonetheless, it is noteworthy that may patients state that they prefer the side effects of VNS to those of medications. In both the epilepsy and depression studies, most patients elected to continue to receive VNS 1 or 2 years after implantation, indicating substantial tolerability.

Conclusion

Starting with ECT, a host of brain stimulation techniques are under development as interventions to treat psychiatric disorders. VNS is differentiated from ECT, TMS, MST, and DBS in being wedded to stimulation of a particular nerve. Furthermore, although the target of stimulation is the brain, stimulation of the vagus nerve occurs outside the brain. Developments in the field of brain stimulation in psychiatry concentrate on spatial refinement and stimulation parameter refinement. TMS, MST, and DBS have as a primary justification the capacity to target specific brain regions or subregions, in contrast to the type of extracranial stimulation associated, for example, with ECT. But even here, work is under way to develop the capacity for focal seizure induction with a standard electrical stimulus. In ongoing work at Columbia, our goal is to develop both ECT and MST so that the emerging information on the relationships of efficacy to dosage and location can be integrated into routine technique. As conducted at present, VNS involves stimulation outside the brain and modulates widespread patterns of brain activity.

The relative lack of specificity is not necessarily a problem. Poor spatial resolution in affecting brain function usually is associated with a poor side-effect profile. Basically, many of the serious side effects of medications are due to their exerting actions in structures or systems distinct from those involved in therapeutic effects (e.g., parkinsonism in patients treated with neuroleptics). However, the side-effect profile, at least as reported by patients, appears especially benign with VNS. Why this is the case is not known, especially because other treatments with anticonvulsant properties, whether physical (e.g., ECT) or pharmacologic, often have the potential for debilitating side effects.

The efficacy of VNS is uncertain. The tantalizing aspect of this intervention is that it appears to improve with time, almost like a fine wine. Many clinicians are convinced that months or years after implantation, patients may have dramatic improvement in seizure frequency or mood state. Unfortunately, this claim of enhanced efficacy with time has never been tested directly but has been mostly inferred from uncontrolled aspects of trials. This is the crux of the matter.

In psychiatry, we are unlikely to recommend VNS or DBS for a "quick fix." Given that an implantation will be performed, clinicians and patients will look for a sustained effect. Unfortunately, all the data pertaining to this issue in epilepsy and depression are naturalistic and confounded. In the naturalistic setting of clinical practice, changes in symptom profiles often trigger changes in treatment regimen, and it is impossible to tell which came first. To determine with confidence that VNS has a role in the treatment of major depression, controlled, randomized trials focusing on long-term effects are clearly needed.

References

Amar AP, DeGiorgio CM, Tarver WB, et al: Long-term multicenter experience with vagus nerve stimulation for intractable partial seizures: results of the XE5 trial. Stereotact Funct Neurosurg 73:104–108, 1999

American Psychiatric Association: Diagnostic and Statistical Manual of Mental Disorders, 4th Edition. Washington, DC, American Psychiatric Association, 1994

Bailey P, Bremer F: A sensory cortical representation of the vagus nerve. J Neurophysiol 1:405–412, 1938

Ben-Menachem E: Vagus nerve stimulation for treatment of seizures? Arch Neurol 55:231–232, 1998

Ben-Menachem E: Vagus nerve stimulation, side effects, and long-term safety. J Clin Neurophysiol 18:415–418, 2001

Ben-Menachem E, Manon-Espaillat R, Ristanovic R, et al: Vagus nerve stimulation for treatment of partial seizures, 1: a controlled study of effect on seizures. First International Vagus Nerve Stimulation Study Group. Epilepsia 35:616–626, 1994

Ben-Menachem E, Hamberger A, Hedner T, et al: Effects of vagus nerve stimulation on amino acids and other metabolites in the CSF of patients with partial seizures. Epilepsy Res 20:221–227, 1995

Binnie CD: Vagus nerve stimulation for epilepsy: a review. Seizure 9:161–169, 2000

Bohning DE, Lomarev MP, Denslow S, et al: Feasibility of vagus nerve stimulation-synchronized blood oxygenation level-dependent functional MRI. Invest Radiol 36:470–479, 2001

Charous SJ, Kempster G, Manders E, et al: The effect of vagal nerve stimulation on voice. Laryngoscope 111:2028–2031, 2001

Clark KB, Smith DC, Hassert DL, et al: Posttraining electrical stimulation of vagal afferents with concomitant vagal efferent inactivation enhances memory storage processes in the rat. Neurobiol Learn Mem 70:364–373, 1998

Clark KB, Naritoku DK, Smith DC, et al: Enhanced recognition memory following vagus nerve stimulation in human subjects. Nat Neurosci 2:94–98, 1999

Dell P, Olson R: Projections "secondaires" mesencéphaliques, diencéphaliques et amygdaliennes des afferences viscérales vagales. CR Soc Biol (Paris) 145:1088–1091, 1951

DeLong MR, Alexander GE, Georgopoulos AP, et al: Role of basal ganglia in limb movements. Hum Neurobiol 2:235–244, 1984

DiMatteo MR, Lepper HS, Croghan TW: Depression is a risk factor for noncompliance with medical treatment: meta-analysis of the effects of anxiety and depression on patient adherence. Arch Intern Med 160:2101–2107, 2000

Dossi RC, Nuñez A, Steriade M: Electrophysiology of a slow (0.5–4 Hz) intrinsic oscillation of cat thalamocortical neurones in vivo. J Physiol 447:215–234, 1992

Drevets WC: Neuroimaging studies of mood disorders. Biol Psychiatry 48:813–829, 2000

Drevets WC, Bogers W, Raichle ME: Functional anatomical correlates of antidepressant drug treatment assessed using PET measures of regional glucose metabolism. Eur Neuropsychopharmacol 12:527–544, 2002

Fromm GH, Amores CY, Thies W: Imipramine in epilepsy. Arch Neurol 27:198–204, 1972

George R, Salinsky M, Kuzniecky R, et al: Vagus nerve stimulation for treatment of partial seizures: 3, long-term follow-up on first 67 patients exiting a controlled study. First International Vagus Nerve Stimulation Study Group. Epilepsia 35:637–643, 1994

George MS, Lisanby SH, Sackeim HA: Transcranial magnetic stimulation: applications in psychiatry. Arch Gen Psychiatry 56:300–311, 1999

George MS, Sackeim HA, Marangell LB, et al: Vagus nerve stimulation: a potential therapy for resistant depression? Psychiatr Clin North Am 23:757–783, 2000a

George MS, Sackeim HA, Rush AJ, et al: Vagus nerve stimulation: a new tool for brain research and therapy. Biol Psychiatry 47:287–295, 2000b

George MS, Rush AJ, Sackeim HA, et al: Vagus nerve stimulation (VNS): utility in neuropsychiatric disorders. Int J Neuropharmacol 6:73–83, 2003

Gieroba ZJ, Blessing WW: Fos-containing neurons in medulla and pons after unilateral stimulation of the afferent abdominal vagus in conscious rabbits. Neuroscience 59:851–858, 1994

Handforth A, DeGiorgio CM, Schachter SC, et al: Vagus nerve stimulation therapy for partial-onset seizures: a randomized active-control trial. Neurology 51:48–55, 1998

Harden CL, Pulver MC, Ravdin LD, et al: A pilot study of mood in epilepsy patients treated with vagus nerve stimulation. Epilepsy Behav 1:93–99, 2000

Haslinger B, Boecker H, Buchel C, et al: Differential modulation of subcortical target and cortex during deep brain stimulation. Neuroimage 18:517–524, 2003

Helmstaedter C, Hoppe C, Elger CE: Memory alterations during acute high-intensity vagus nerve stimulation. Epilepsy Res 47:37–42, 2001

Henry TR: Functional imaging studies of epilepsy therapies. Adv Neurol 83:305–317, 2000

Henry TR: Therapeutic mechanisms of vagus nerve stimulation. Neurology 59 (6, suppl 4):S3–14, 2002

Henry TR, Bakay RA, Votaw JR, et al: Brain blood flow alterations induced by therapeutic vagus nerve stimulation in partial epilepsy, I: acute effects at high and low levels of stimulation. Epilepsia 39:983–990, 1998

Henry TR, Votaw JR, Pennell PB, et al: Acute blood flow changes and efficacy of vagus nerve stimulation in partial epilepsy. Neurology 52:1166–1173, 1999

Hoppe C, Helmstaedter C, Scherrmann J, et al: No evidence for cognitive side effects after 6 months of vagus nerve stimulation in epilepsy patients. 2:351–356, 2001

Ko D, Heck C, Grafton S, et al: Vagus nerve stimulation activates central nervous system structures in epileptic patients during PET H$_2$(15)O blood flow imaging. Neurosurgery 39:426–430, 1996

Krahl SE, Clark KB, Smith DC, et al: Locus coeruleus lesions suppress the seizure-attenuating effects of vagus nerve stimulation. Epilepsia 39:709–714, 1998

Labar D: Vagus nerve stimulation for intractable epilepsy in children. Dev Med Child Neurol 42:496–499, 2000

Labar D, Murphy J, Tecoma E: Vagus nerve stimulation for medication-resistant generalized epilepsy. E04 VNS Study Group. Neurology 52:1510–1512, 1999

Lisanby SH, Schlaepfer TE, Fisch HU, et al: Magnetic seizure therapy of major depression. Arch Gen Psychiatry 58:303–305, 2001

Lisanby SH, Luber B, Schlaepfer TE, et al: Safety and feasibility of magnetic seizure therapy (MST) in major depression: randomized comparison with electroconvulsive therapy. Neuropsychopharmacology 28:1852–1865, 2003

MacLean PD: The Triune Brain in Evolution: Role in Paleocerebral Functions. New York, Plenum, 1990

Marangell LB, Rush AJ, George MS, et al: Vagus nerve stimulation (VNS) for major depressive episodes: one year outcomes. Biol Psychiatry 51:280–287, 2002

Mayberg HS: Modulating dysfunctional limbic-cortical circuits in depression: towards development of brain-based algorithms for diagnosis and optimised treatment. Br Med Bull 65:193–207, 2003

McCall WV, Reboussin DM, Weiner RD, et al: Titrated moderately suprathreshold vs fixed high-dose right unilateral electroconvulsive therapy: acute antidepressant and cognitive effects. Arch Gen Psychiatry 57:438–444, 2000

McLachlan RS: Vagus nerve stimulation for treatment of seizures? Arch Neurol 55:232–233, 1998

Morris GL 3rd, Mueller WM: Long-term treatment with vagus nerve stimulation in patients with refractory epilepsy. The Vagus Nerve Stimulation Study Group E01–E05. Neurology 53:1731–1735, 1999

Murphy JV: Left vagal nerve stimulation in children with medically refractory epilepsy. The Pediatric VNS Study Group. J Pediatr 134:563–566, 1999

Nagarajan L, Walsh P, Gregory P, et al: VNS therapy in clinical practice in children with refractory epilepsy. Acta Neurol Scand 105:13–17, 2002

Narayanan JT, Watts R, Haddad N, et al: Cerebral activation during vagus nerve stimulation: a functional MR study. Epilepsia 43:1509–1514, 2002

Naritoku DK, Terry WJ, Helfert RH: Regional induction of fos immunoreactivity in the brain by anticonvulsant stimulation of the vagus nerve. Epilepsy Res 22:53–62, 1995

Nobler MS, Sackeim HA, Prohovnik I, et al: Regional cerebral blood flow in mood disorders, III: treatment and clinical response. Arch Gen Psychiatry 51:884–897, 1994

Nobler MS, Roose SP, Prohovnik I, et al: Regional cerebral blood flow in mood disorders, V: effects of antidepressant medication in late-life depression. Am J Geriatr Psychiatry 8:289–296, 2000

Nobler MS, Oquendo MA, Kegeles LS, et al: Decreased regional brain metabolism after ECT. Am J Psychiatry 158:305–308, 2001

Paus T, Jech R, Thompson CJ, et al: Dose-dependent reduction of cerebral blood flow during rapid-rate transcranial magnetic stimulation of the human sensorimotor cortex. J Neurophysiol 79:1102–1107, 1998

Penry JK, Dean JC: Prevention of intractable partial seizures by intermittent vagal stimulation in humans: preliminary results. Epilepsia 31 (suppl 2):S40–S43, 1990

Ramsay RE, Uthman BM, Augustinsson LE, et al: Vagus nerve stimulation for treatment of partial seizures: 2, safety, side effects, and tolerability. First International Vagus Nerve Stimulation Study Group. Epilepsia 35:627–636, 1994

Ring HA, White S, Costa DC, et al: A SPECT study of the effect of vagal nerve stimulation on thalamic activity in patients with epilepsy. Seizure 9:380–384, 2000

Rush AJ, George MS, Sackeim HA, et al: Vagus nerve stimulation (VNS) for treatment-resistant depressions: a multicenter study. Biol Psychiatry 47:276–286, 2000

Rutecki P: Anatomical, physiological, and theoretical basis for the antiepileptic effect of vagus nerve stimulation. Epilepsia 31 (suppl 2):S1–S6, 1990

Sackeim HA: Magnetic stimulation therapy and ECT. Convuls Ther 10:255–258, 1994

Sackeim HA: The anticonvulsant hypothesis of the mechanisms of action of ECT: current status. J ECT 15:5–26, 1999

Sackeim HA: Repetitive transcranial magnetic stimulation: what are the next steps? Biol Psychiatry 48:959–961, 2000

Sackeim HA: The definition and meaning of treatment-resistant depression. J Clin Psychiatry 62 (suppl 16):10–17, 2001

Sackeim HA, Decina P, Prohovnik I, et al: Anticonvulsant and antidepressant properties of electroconvulsive therapy: a proposed mechanism of action. Biol Psychiatry 18:1301–1310, 1983

Sackeim HA, Prudic J, Devanand DP, et al: Effects of stimulus intensity and electrode placement on the efficacy and cognitive effects of electroconvulsive therapy. N Engl J Med 328:839–846, 1993

Sackeim HA, Luber B, Katzman GP, et al: The effects of electroconvulsive therapy on quantitative electroencephalograms: relationship to clinical outcome. Arch Gen Psychiatry 53:814–824, 1996

Sackeim HA, Luber B, Moeller JR, et al: Electrophysiological correlates of the adverse cognitive effects of electroconvulsive therapy. J ECT 16:110–120, 2000a

Sackeim HA, Prudic J, Devanand DP, et al: A prospective, randomized, double-blind comparison of bilateral and right unilateral electroconvulsive therapy at different stimulus intensities. Arch Gen Psychiatry 57:425–434, 2000b

Sackeim HA, Haskett RF, Mulsant BH, et al: Continuation pharmacotherapy in the prevention of relapse following electroconvulsive therapy: a randomized controlled trial. JAMA 285:1299–1307, 2001a

Sackeim HA, Keilp JG, Rush AJ, et al: The effects of vagus nerve stimulation on cognitive performance in patients with treatment-resistant depression. Neuropsychiatry Neuropsychol Behav Neurol 14:53–62, 2001b

Sackeim HA, Rush AJ, George MS, et al: Vagus nerve stimulation (VNS) for treatment-resistant depression: efficacy, side effects, and predictors of outcome. Neuropsychopharmacology 25:713–728, 2001c

Shukla S, Mukherjee S, Decina P: Lithium in the treatment of bipolar disorders associated with epilepsy: an open study. J Clin Psychopharmacol 8:201–204, 1988

Sjogren MJ, Hellstrom PT, Jonsson MA, et al: Cognition-enhancing effect of vagus nerve stimulation in patients with Alzheimer's disease: a pilot study. J Clin Psychiatry 63:972–980, 2002

Steriade M: Cellular substrates of brain rhythms, in Electroencephalography: Basic Principles, Clinical Applications, and Related Fields, 3rd Edition. Edited by Lopes da Silva FH. Baltimore, MD, Williams & Wilkins, 1994, pp 27–62

Thielscher A, Kammer T: Linking physics with physiology in TMS: a sphere field model to determine the cortical stimulation site in TMS. Neuroimage 17:1117–1130, 2002

Vagus Nerve Stimulation Study Group: A randomized controlled trial of chronic vagus nerve stimulation for treatment of medically intractable seizures. Neurology 45:224–230, 1995

Van Laere K, Vonck K, Boon P, et al: Vagus nerve stimulation in refractory epilepsy: SPECT activation study. J Nucl Med 41:1145–1154, 2000

Van Laere K, Vonck K, Boon P, et al: Perfusion SPECT changes after acute and chronic vagus nerve stimulation in relation to prestimulus condition and long-term clinical efficacy. J Nucl Med 43:733–744, 2002

Vesper J, Klostermann F, Stockhammer F, et al: Results of chronic sub-thalamic nucleus stimulation for Parkinson's disease: a 1-year follow-up study. Surg Neurol 57:306–311, 2002

Vitek JL: Mechanisms of deep brain stimulation: excitation or inhibition. Mov Disord 17 (suppl 3):S69–S72, 2002

Vonck K, Boon P, Van Laere K, et al: Acute single photon emission computed tomographic study of vagus nerve stimulation in refractory epilepsy. Epilepsia 41:601–609, 2000

Walker BR, Easton A, Gale K: Regulation of limbic motor seizures by GABA and glutamate transmission in nucleus tractus solitarius. Epilepsia 40:1051–1057, 1999

Woodbury DM, Woodbury JW: Effects of vagal stimulation on experimentally induced seizures in rats. Epilepsia 31 (suppl 2):S7–S19, 1990

Woodbury JW, Woodbury DM: Vagal stimulation reduces the severity of maximal electroshock seizures in intact rats: use of a cuff electrode for stimulating and recording. Pacing Clin Electrophysiol 14:94–107, 1991

Yousfi-Malki M, Puizillout JJ: Induction of Fos-like protein in neurons of the medulla oblongata after electrical stimulation of the vagus nerve in anesthetized rabbit. Brain Res 635:317–322, 1994

Zabara J: Peripheral control of hypersynchronous discharge in epilepsy. Electroencephalogr Clin Neurophysiol 61 (suppl): S162, 1985a

Zabara J: Time course of seizure control to brief, repetitive stimuli (abstract). Epilepsia 26:518, 1985b

Zabara J: Inhibition of experimental seizures in canines by repetitive vagal stimulation. Epilepsia 33:1005–1012, 1992

Index

*Page numbers printed in **boldface** type refer to tables or figures.*

Electroconvulsive therapy (ECT)
(continued)
improved tolerability of,
through MST, 69, 72
long-term risks in, 9
MST vs., 13, 74–75, 89–91
rTMS vs., 14
risk/benefit ratio, 72–73
side effects, xvi, 72– 73, 85–87,
86
spatial imprecision of, 74
Electroencephalographic (EEG)
measures
and ECT, 73
and MST vs. ECT, 87
and rTMS in auditory
hallucinations of
schizophrenia, 34, 35
Electromagnetic fields, high-
frequency, 10
Epilepsy. *See also* Seizures
and brain regions affected by
of VNS, 110
DBS for, 54
imaging studies, 109–110
treatment-resistant, and VNS,
117–119
VNS for, 108, 115, 116, 119–121,
134
Essential tremor. *See* Tremor,
essential
Ethical issues in DBS, 60–62
Extinction process, 45–46

Faraday, Michael, 2
FDA. *See* U.S. Food and Drug
Administration
FDG (fluorodeoxyglucose) PET, 27
Figure-eight coil. *See* Coils
Fluorodeoxyglucose (FDG) PET,
27

Fluoxetine for obsessive-
compulsive disorder, 29
fMRI (functional magnetic
resonance imaging), 40–41,
45
Focal brain stimulation, xvi–xvii,
12, 13, 15, 74, 79, 80, 87–89,
100, 104, 135
Focal dystonia, 25
Focal seizures, ability to induce,
xvi
Food and Drug Administration.
See U.S. Food and Drug
Administration
Freezing behavior, 45
Frequency (Hz), for rTMS,
23–25
Functional magnetic resonance
imaging (fMRI), 40–41, 45.
See also BOLD

GABA (γ-aminobutyric acid), 110,
123
Globus pallidus, 101, **102–103,**
104
Glutamate, 110, 123

Hallucinations, xvi. *See also*
Auditory hallucinations
Hamilton Rating Scale for
Depression (Ham-D) scores
and MST, 85
and TMS, 11, 13
and VNS, 124, 125, 131
Handwriting impairment
(writer's cramp), 25–26
Headache, as side effect, 9
Hippocampus
and plasticity, 81–83
and spatial distribution of
induced seizures, 79

procedure for, 105–106
pulse amplitude for, 115–116
purpose of, 105
response rates to, **120**
for seizure control in epilepsy,
    110
    study E01, 119
    study E02, 119
    study E03, 117–119
    study E04, 119
    study E05, 115, 117–119
    trial E03, 115
and sham stimulation, 129,
    130, 131
side effects of, 113, 115,
    133–135
stimulus parameters for, 113,
    114, 115, 116
studies of, 115, 117–119, 126,
    135

surgical implantation for,
    111–112
waiting period after, 112
and treatment adherence, 112
for treatment-resistant
    epilepsy, 117–119
Valproate, 122
Ventral anterior/ventral lateral
    thalamic nuclei, 101, **102–103**
Vertigo, 2
VNS. *See* Vagus nerve stimulation
Voice alteration, as side effect,
    115, 122, 128, 133, 135
Wernicke's area in schizophrenia,
    33, 40, 45
Writer's cramp, 25–26

Yale-Brown Obsessive
    Compulsive Scale (YBOCS),
    29